Guides to Clinical
Aspiration Biopsy

Breast

Guides to Clinical Aspiration Biopsy

Series Editor: Tilde S. Kline, M.D.

Prostate
Tilde S. Kline, M.D.

Thyroid
Sudha R. Kini, M.D.

Retroperitoneum and Intestine
Kenneth C. Suen, M.B., B.S., F.R.C.P.(C)

Lung, Pleura and Mediastinum
Liang-Che Tao, M.D., F.C.A.P., F.R.C.P.(C)

Head and Neck
Ali H. Qizilbash, M.B., B.S., F.R.C.P.(C)
J. Edward M. Young, M.D., F.R.C.S.(C)

Liver and Pancreas
Denise Frias-Hidvegi, M.D., F.I.A.C.

Breast
Tilde S. Kline, M.D.
Irwin K. Kline, M.D.

Guides to Clinical Aspiration Biopsy

Breast

Tilde S. Kline, M.D.

Associate Pathologist
Chief, Division of Cytology
Lankenau Hospital
Philadelphia, Pennsylvania

Professor of Pathology
Jefferson Medical College of Thomas Jefferson University
Philadelphia, Pennsylvania

Irwin K. Kline, M.D.

Chairman, Department of Pathology
Lankenau Hospital
Philadelphia, Pennsylvania

Professor of Pathology
Jefferson Medical College of Thomas Jefferson University
Philadelphia, Pennsylvania

IGAKU-SHOIN   New York • Tokyo

Typesetting by Achorn Graphic Services, Inc. in Garamond
Printing and Binding by Arcata Graphics/Halliday

Published and distributed by

IGAKU-SHOIN Medical Publishers, Inc.
1140 Avenue of the Americas, New York, N.Y.   10036

IGAKU-SHOIN Ltd.,
5-24-3 Hongo, Bunkyo-ku, Tokyo

Library of Congress Cataloging-in-Publication Data

Kline, Tilde S., 1931–
    Breast / Tilde S. Kline, Irwin K. Kline.
        p.   cm.—(Guides to clinical aspiration biopsy)
    Includes index.
    1. Breast—Biopsy, Needle.   2. Breast—Diseases—Diagnosis.
3. Breast—Cancer—Diagnosis.   4. Diagnosis, Cytologic.   I. Kline,
Irwin K.   II. Title.   III. Series.
RG493.5.B56K58   1989
618.1'907'58—dc19   89-1938

ISBN: 0-89640-159-6 (New York)
ISBN: 4-260-14159-7 (Tokyo)

Printed and bound in U.S.A.

10 9 8 7 6 5 4 3 2 1

Preface

This monograph, the seventh in the series *Guides to Clinical Aspiration Biopsy,* has been written to meet the needs of the pathologist, cytotechnologist, and clinician in the diagnosis of breast disease by aspiration biopsy cytology. In our institution, this modality has altered the approach to lesions of the breast. Formerly, virtually every breast biopsy entailed frozen section diagnosis. Additionally, in some unfortunate cases, watchful waiting preceded biopsy. Currently, almost every breast lesion is examined initially by fine-needle aspiration biopsy, and decision-making is based on the results. At the same time, specimens are aspirated from suspicious lesions for preliminary evaluation of hormone receptors. In the future, reports indicate that prognoses based on cytophotometry and flow cytometry will be made by fine-needle aspiration biopsy. The views presented here are based on practical experience over the years, as well as on information gained from extensive review of the literature.

This monograph embodies the philosophy of the series. Cytomorphology and histology are considered together. Tables are presented for rapid orientation and interpretation. Although different techniques are set forth, the biopsy specimen procured by the clinician and prepared according to the method of Papanicolaou is stressed. This approach has been used successfully in our institution for 20 years. The photographs emphasize the pattern approach to aspiration biopsy cytology. Therefore, many low-magnification views precede those displaying cellular details. Comparative cytomorphologic features of allied lesions are depicted for differential diagnosis.

Grateful acknowledgment is due to our colleagues in the preparation and presentation of this work. We are especially indebted to our associates Vaidehi Kannan, Ilona Ring, Joseph Cooper, and Frank McBrearty, who gave freely of their knowledge in collection of the data. The cooperation and secretarial skill of Michelle Darby and Delores Pascale have been invaluable. We also wish to thank Carolyn Lachowicz for her reading and criticism of the manuscript. Other persons from the laboratory who presented many helpful suggestions include Suzanne Kent, Mary Cahalan, Maryann Davis, Linda Muzroll, Claire Sims, and Cecilia Gallagher. Special thanks are due to Tess Jennifer Kline and Janine Pilon for their photographic assistance and to Marie Norton for utilizing her outstanding skills as a reference librarian in our behalf.

Tilde S. Kline, M.D.
Irwin K. Kline, M.D.

To our children and enlarged family
Tonie, Doug, Jody, Cathy, Tess, Stephan, and Sebastian

Foreword

"It is the mind which is really alive and sees things, yet it hardly sees anything without preliminary instruction" (Charcot).

For a procedure to be assimilated into the core of patient management, it must:

1. influence the decision-making process;
2. be cost effective;
3. be replicable in a variety of clinical situations.

Aspiration biopsy cytology (ABC) of the breast certainly fulfills these criteria and is now an established and time-tested element in the diagnosis of breast pathology.

This volume is a distillate of almost two decades of intensive experience involving over 14,000 aspirates from the breast. While principally intended as a text of cytomorphology for cytologists and cytopathologists, it contains material of considerable value for the clinician. It is important for the cytopathologist to know something of the patient in question; it is equally important for the clinician to know something of the language and problems of aspiration biopsy cytology. It is through this mutual effort that ABC fulfills its promise to dispel indecision and hasten therapy in malignant disease. Dr. Kline has achieved her instructional goal in making aspiration biopsy as replicable as possible in a wide variety of clinical situations.

Hunter S. Neal, M.D., F.A.C.S.
Chairman, Department of Surgery
Lankenau Hospital
Philadelphia, PA

Contributors

Christopher P. Holroyde, M.D.
Director, Oncology, Cancer Treatment Center
Lankenau Hospital
Philadelphia, Pennsylvania
and
Associate Professor of Medicine
Jefferson Medical College of Thomas Jefferson University
Philadelphia, Pennsylvania

Lydia Pleotis Howell, M.D.
Assistant Clinical Professor of Pathology
University of California, Davis Medical Center
Sacramento, California

Albert A. Keshgegian, M.D., Ph.D.
Associate Director, Department of Pathology
Bryn Mawr Hospital
Bryn Mawr, Pennsylvania
and
Adjunct Associate Professor of Pathology and Laboratory Medicine
School of Medicine, University of Pennsylvania
Philadelphia, Pennsylvania

Karen K. Lindfors, M.D.
Assistant Professor of Radiology
Chief of Mammography
University of California, Davis Medical Center
Sacramento, California

Joel Lundy, M.D.
Director, Surgical Oncology
Winthrop-University Hospital
Mineola, New York
and
Associate Professor of Surgery
State University of New York School of Medicine
Stony Brook, New York

Sally Rosen, M.D.
Deputy Director, Cytology
Associate Professor of Pathology
Temple University Hospital
Philadelphia, Pennsylvania

Robert D. Smink, Jr., M.D.
Chief, Division of General Surgery
Lankenau Hospital
Philadelphia, Pennsylvania
and
Clinical Assistant Professor of Surgery
Jefferson Medical College of Thomas Jefferson University
Philadelphia, Pennsylvania

Kaighn Smith, M.D.
Chairman, Department of Obstetrics and Gynecology
Lankenau Hospital
Philadelphia, Pennsylvania
and
Professor of Obstetrics and Gynecology
Jefferson Medical College of Thomas Jefferson University
Philadelphia, Pennsylvania

Contents

Key to abbreviations

ABC	Aspiration Biopsy Cytology
NAB	Needle Aspiration Biopsy

1

Introduction

INTRODUCTION

Recent years have ushered in a new era for diagnosis and treatment of breast carcinoma. The growth of fine-needle aspiration biopsy [NAB (the biopsy procedure)] has paralleled these changes, which have been mirrored in our own practice. Initially, at our institution, this biopsy was used exclusively for preliminary interpretation of palpable masses. Within several years, the focus had altered. In many cases NAB was substituted for tissue biopsy, or else the latter became an ambulatory procedure. These two complementary procedures have gradually altered the profile of breast surgery. Frozen section diagnosis of breast lesions followed by definitive surgery for carcinoma has been almost eliminated in our institution (see Chapter 8).

Mammograms are shifting the emphasis for detection of breast disease by pinpointing smaller and smaller lesions. To turn these shadows into substance, aspiration biopsy cytology [ABC (the aspirated cells)] is assuming an expanding role. Initiated in Sweden more than a decade ago,[3] its implementation by NAB during the localization procedure in the radiology suite has finally attracted the attention of the medical profession in the United States (see Chapter 10). The simple "scouting needle" procedure for rapid office evaluation of mammographic abnormalities, devised by Hunter S. Neal, has also become an effective preliminary device (see the "Biopsy Procedure" in Chapter 3 and Chapter 8). The so-called high-risk lesions of atypical hyperplasia, in situ lobular carcinoma, and intraductal carcinoma are being uncovered by these procedures and are addressed in Chapter 12.

Today the therapeutic options for breast carcinoma are varied. Lumpectomy has added a new dimension to treatment. The follow-up of these patients has grown even more critical, necessitating immediate evaluation of abnormalities in or near the surgical margins of excision. NAB can be an optimum tool for the oncologist (see the section on "The Internist-Oncologist and NAB" in Chapter 8 and Chapter 9).

The role of estrogen and progesterone receptors has become increasingly important in the selection of therapy. The application of immunocytochemical techniques to ABC has evolved into a practical procedure for the cytology laboratory. Studies indicate the potential of these agents applied to the aspirates not only for immunoassays of estrogen and progesterone receptors[15] but also for tumor markers[18,25] (see the section on "The Surgeon and NAB" in Chapter 8 and Chapter 9).

New modalities in the diagnostic armamentarium, developed in the research laboratory, will soon be utilized in the general cytology laboratory. One of these is flow cytometry, with its application to treatment and prognosis. NAB can provide samples for these proliferating techniques (see Chapter 12).

Finally, NAB is not in competition with excisional biopsy. Many times, however, this simple, cost-effective, fine-needle office procedure can be substituted for the latter modality, limiting the spiraling cost of the operating room. Nonetheless, NAB should be used neither to substitute for clinical judgment nor to exclude an indicated histopathologic biopsy.

HISTORY

"One can never feel quite sure regarding the nature of palpable abnormalities in the female breast without a biopsy, but for practical reasons excision biopsy cannot be used unrestrictedly." So stated the Swedish clinician Söderström[35] in his 1966 monograph, *Fine Needle Aspiration Biopsy*. He continued, "I dared attempt it as a routine method only after my surgical colleagues agreed to regard all negative reports as no reports at all and to manage the patients accordingly. The results proved satisfactory, . . . [and the biopsies detected] a number of early cancers with clinically trifling findings which might otherwise have remained undetected." These words summarized the importance of the technique, pioneered by the clinician Martin and the technologist Ellis in 1930,[26] with the able assistance of the pathologist Stewart. Their initial study included 6 breast tumors, which rose to 500 by 1933 and prompted Stewart[36] to write, "The procedure is so simple and useful that at the present time almost every breast lesion that presents itself in the breast clinic is aspirated if the least possibility of mammary carcinoma is considered." He recommended it for patients to be treated by radiation alone, for those developing a tumor during pregnancy and lactation, to confirm the diagnosis of tumor, to rule out contralateral carcinoma, to differentiate carcinoma from suppurative mastitis, to diagnose deep-seated nodules, and to distinguish necrosis from recurrent breast carcinoma.

Despite Stewart's eloquence, over the next 25 years only rare publications confirmed the efficacy of this approach.[5,10,31] Then Papanicolaou et al.[29] in 1958 recorded the use of the procedure on 94 patients, and by 1959 Cornillot and Verhaeghe[6,7] had emphasized its safety and simplicity by the demonstration of 500 cases. In Sweden by 1970, Franzén and Zajicek and colleagues[12,39] had completed a study of 2,111 patients. With this large data bank, aspiration biopsy has developed into an important tool for examination of all breast masses. A number of investigators, notable in its flowering, are cited in subsequent sections, and there have been two monographs on the subject. In the first, published in 1978, the German Schöndörf[32] utilized the European technique and described his findings on 2,778 breast lesions. More recently, Oertel,[27] also a fervid proponent of the single-operator approach and the Romanovsky technique, published the results of her own experience with 3,602 mammary aspirates.

NAB was inaugurated at Lankenau Hospital in 1970 by Hunter S. Neal, now Chairman of Surgery. From its beginnings at our institution, the team approach has been practiced, whereby clinicians have performed the biopsy and the cytopathologist has interpreted specimens prepared according to the method of Papanicolaou.[19-22] In this manner, we have accumulated more than 14,000 cases. In the following pages our findings are presented, as well as those from the literature, all reflecting the ever-increasing interest in and wealth of material on this subject.

INDICATIONS AND ADVANTAGES

NAB should be adopted as a standard clinical procedure for the evaluation of all palpable breast masses. It can also be used for nonpalpable lesions (see the section on "Scouting NAB" in Chapter 2 and Chapter 10). This technique is indicated for:

1. Evaluation of multiple nodules.
2. Separation of a cyst from a solid tumor, with therapeutic drainage.
3. Distinction between mastitis and inflammatory carcinoma.
4. Evaluation of new masses following therapy.
5. Differentiation of lesions in the tail of the breast (i.e., lymph node and breast disease).
6. Evaluation of vague masses and painful nontumorous areas.
7. Assay of hormonal receptors.

The advantages of this procedure are multifold. NAB provides a prompt, cost-effective,[1,11,24] safe procedure, appropriate for office evaluation, that finds ready patient acceptance. Positive ABC in experienced hands can be substituted for excisional biopsy and provides:

1. Psychologic preparation of the patient.
2. Discussion of therapeutic options, aided by the cytomorphologic impression of the tumor type.
3. Effective utilization of operating room time.
4. Planned surgical approach for either lumpectomy or mastectomy.
5. Assistance in staging (see Chapter 9).

LIMITATIONS AND COMPLICATIONS

There are no contraindications to NAB of the breast. The size or depth of the lesion may be limiting factors without radiographic guidance. Schöndorf,[32] however, recovered malignant cells from tiny lesions in 18 of 19 cases. In another series of tumors <1.0 cm encompassing both palpable lesions and those requiring the scouting needle technique (see Chapter 2), we[33] detected tumor cells in 9 of 32 cases and interpreted 8 more as suspicious. Some[34] suggest that mammography should be delayed for 2 weeks following NAB to prevent possible misinterpretation because of focal hemorrhage.

Possible complications are remote. Hematoma formation can be prevented or alleviated by applying firm pressure immediately at the time of biopsy. Infection has not proved consequential. A rarely reported complication is pneumothorax.[4,13] Penetration of the fine needle through the breast into the thorax has occurred only twice among our more than 14,000 cases.

The much discussed tumor spread by the fine needle is almost a myth. Data from postoperative patients 5 and 10 years after diagnostic NAB, in contrast to those without NAB, disclosed a similar survival.[2,30] In fact, a projected study by the National Surgical Adjuvant Breast Project Group will rely on diagnosis by NAB followed by preoperative chemotherapy before definitive surgery.

CONTRASTS: ABC AND EXFOLIATIVE CYTOLOGY

Interpretation of ABC both resembles and differs from that of exfoliative cytology. The former is based on pattern, whereas the latter is based on individual cell examination. The scanning lens ($\times 2.5$) is indicated for the initial and final examinations of only ABC. To facilitate this inspection, neither cytopathologists nor cytotechnologists use the mechanical stage in our institution.

Diagnostic parameters for ABC deviate from those for exfoliative cytology (Table 1.1). The three most important judgmental criteria are (1) cellularity, (2) dyshesion ("disordered cell adherence" [*Dorland's Medical Dictionary*, 27th ed.]), and (3) monomorphism (one cell form), by contrast to the altered nuclear/cytoplasmic ratio and hyperchromasia of exfoliated cells. Criteria common to both modalities include anisonucleosis (unequal nuclear size), nuclear membrane irregularity, and eosinophilic macronucleoli (>1.25 μm in diameter). A sanguineous, inflammatory diathesis, significant in exfoliative cytology, plays a lesser role in the interpretation of ABC. Although each criterion may not be in evidence in a single case or specific type of tumor, the majority will be found.

The aspirate from a benign lesion frequently is cell poor. Cells form large, cohesive, uniform groups. Polymorphism (multiple forms) is common, cell borders are distinct, and nuclear membranes are regular.

TABLE 1.1. ABC Diagnostic Parameters

Features*	Malignant Tumors	Benign Lesions
Cellularity	+3	+1
Dyshesion	+3	±
Monomorphism	+2	−
Nuclear membrane irregularity	+2	−
Anisonucleosis	+3	+1
Eosinophilic macronucleoli	+2	±

*No single feature is pathognomonic of either malignant or benign disease.

Thus, it is apparent that a bridge must be traversed from the interpretation of exfoliative cytology to the interpretation of ABC. Upon application of these special diagnostic criteria to each specimen, ABC interpretation usually is swift and accurate.

DIAGNOSTIC PHRASEOLOGY

In our laboratory, ABC is reported similarly to tissue sections whenever possible. A benign diagnosis includes the terms "fibrocystic change," "fibroadenoma," "papilloma," and the other entities described in Chapter 5. In certain cases, particularly those associated with fibrocystic change, the cell population is limited. In these instances, a descriptive rather than a definitive interpretation reveals the quantity and type of cells. We commence with "No malignant tumor cells seen" and add the following qualifiers:

1. "Relatively sparse aspirate."
2. "A few benign epithelial cells."
3. "Fibroadipose tissue."
4. "? Representative."

With the use of the scouting needle, we add:

5. "? Target contact."
6. "Microcalcifications present (or absent)."

For terminology related to benign cysts, see the section on "Benign Cysts" in Chapter 4.

An "unsatisfactory" diagnosis is issued for specimens that are inadequate for interpretation (see Table 2.3). Therefore, decision-making on the basis of such an aspirate, which is equivalent to no biopsy, is impossible. This "nondiagnosis" is issued because of:

1. Insufficient numbers of cells for interpretation.
2. Poorly preserved cells.
3. Epithelial cells obscured by inflammation, blood, or debris.

A "suspicious" interpretation is a meaningful diagnosis, and immediate excisional biopsy is urged for these cases. This interpretation is made because of:

1. Lack of some of the criteria for malignancy.
2. Insufficient numbers of abnormal cells.
3. Inadequate preservation of abnormal cells.
4. Abnormal cells which cannot be categorized.

A "positive" diagnosis is equivalent to excisional biopsy in our institution, and leads directly to patient counseling and therapy. It is based on the criteria for malignancy reflected in adequate numbers of well-preserved cells. It is made by using the team approach (see Chapter 2) and is discussed with the clinician prior to transmission of the written report. A positive diagnosis includes the classification and the degree of tumor differentiation whenever possible.

STATISTICS

The sensitivity of NAB in studies with a minimum of 500 cases generally ranges from 89 to 98 percent (Table 1.2). It is influenced both by the nature of the institution and by the technique. In large cancer referral centers, prescreened patients offer the greatest yield of malignant tumors. The highest accuracy has been reported from institutions where a single individual obtains and interprets the biopsy specimen.

In our laboratory, the sensitivity rises from 90 to 94 percent upon exclusion of nonpalpable masses sampled by the scouting needle.[33] The predictive value of our positive reports is 100 percent, an essential ingredient when this interpretation is equivalent to excisional tissue biopsy. Nevertheless, in programs such as ours, where most breast lesions are screened by NAB, a suspicious interpretation is meaningful: It carries the recommendation of immediate tissue biopsy, since less than 2 percent of our aspirates from benign lesions are so interpreted.[16]

Statistics on the performance of the scouting needle, described in Chapter 2, merit consideration. From a current prospective study in our institution of 221 patients with nonpalpable mammographic abnormalities, there were 42 verified carcinomas. Of these, 43 percent were interpreted by ABC as positive and 14 percent as suspicious, findings indicative of immediate surgical intervention. While the false-negative results are considerably lower than acceptable levels, these encouraging results suggest that the scouting needle be the initial investigative tool for

TABLE 1.2. Breast Carcinoma: Statistics from the Literature

Author	Total Series	ABC, Malignant Tumors*			
		Malignant	Suspicious	Benign	Sensitivity†
Cornillot and Verhaeghe[7]	500	215/237 (91%)	—	22 (9%)	91%
Deschenes et al.[8]	1,478	92/114 (81%)	13 (11%)	9 (8%)	91%
Eisenberg et al.[9]	1,874	1,050/1,389 (76%)	268 (19%)	71 (5%)	94%
Frable[11]	853	269/325 (83%)	29 (9%)	27 (8%)	91%
Halevy et al.[14]	1,953	312/355 (88%)	21 (6%)	22 (6%)	93%
Kline et al.[17]	2,623	257/324 (80%)	37 (12%)	30 (8%)	90%‡
Koivuniemi[23]	1,270	138/188 (73%)	33 (18%)	17 (9%)	89%
Oertel[27]	3,602	685/857 (80%)	122 (14%)	50 (6%)	94%
Palombini et al.[28]	1,956	446/485 (92%)	24 (5%)	15 (3%)	97%
Schöndörf[32]	2,519	283/307 (92%)	18 (6%)	6 (2%)	98%
Young et al.[37]	553	106/134 (79%)	21 (16%)	7 (5%)	94%
Zajdela et al.[38]	6,400	3,081/3,348 (92%)	119 (4%)	148 (4%)	95%
Zajicek et al.[39]	2,111	823/1,068 (77%)	156 (15%)	89 (8%)	90%

*Satisfactory specimens only

†Sensitivity $= \dfrac{\text{True Positive}}{\text{True Positive} + \text{False Negative}} \times 100\%$.

‡Includes both palpable and nonpalpable masses.

mammographic lesions, bolstered by the critical surgeon–radiologist–pathologist partnership.

The majority of false-negative results among experienced personnel are elicited by scirrhous neoplasms, notably the infiltrating lobular carcinoma (see Chapters 6 and 7). Radiation fibrosis may similarly affect evaluation of recurrent tumor (see Chapter 9). The size and locations of the neoplasms can be restrictive. In our series of minimal carcinomas, 47 percent were not penetrated by the fine needle.[33]

False-positive results are a dreaded complication, hopefully to be avoided entirely. False-suspicious findings can never be totally eliminated and are discussed in the following chapters. Unsatisfactory reports, equivalent to no diagnosis whatsoever, are unavoidable to some extent but can be limited by reliable biopsy performance (see the section on "Diagnostic Phraseology" in this chapter and Table 2.2).

REFERENCES

1. Adye B, Jolly PC, Bauermeister DE: The role of fine-needle aspiration in the management of solid breast masses. *Arch Surg* 123:37–39, 1988.

2. Berg JW, Robbins GF: A late look at the safety of aspiration biopsy. *Cancer* 15:826–827, 1962.

3. Bolmgren J, Jacobson B, Nordenström B: Stereotaxic instrument for needle biopsy of the mamma. *Am J Roentgenol* 129:121–125, 1977.

4. Brown JR (ed): Iatrogenic traumatic pneumothorax. *Patient Rx Newsletter* Vol. 4, 1982.

5. Budd JW: Evaluation of needle aspiration technic in breast lesions. *Radiology* 52:502–505, 1949.

6. Cornillot M, Verhaeghe M: Confrontation clinique et cytologique dans les tumeurs de sein. *Cancérologie* 2:204–214, 1955.

7. Cornillot M, Verhaeghe M: Données cytologiques des les ponctions de tumeurs du sein. *Pathol Biol* 7:793–802, 1959.

8. Deschenes L, Fabia J, Meisels A, et al: Fine needle aspiration biopsy in the management of palpable breast lesions. *Can J Surg* 21:417–419, 1978.

9. Eisenberg AJ, Hajdu SI, Wilhelmus J, Melamed MR, Kinne D: Preoperative aspiration cytology of breast tumors. *Acta Cytol* 30:135–146, 1986.

10. Fleming RM: Cytological studies in lesions of the breast. *South Med J* 48:74–78, 1955.

11. Frable WJ: Needle aspiration of the breast. *Cancer* 53:671–676, 1984.

12. Franzén S, Zajicek J: Aspiration biopsy in diagnosis of palpable lesions of the breast. *Acta Radiol* 7:241–262, 1968.

13. Goodson WH III, Malman R, Miller TR: Three year follow-up of benign fine-needle aspiration biopsies of the breast. *Am J Surg* 154:58–61, 1987.

14. Halevy A, Reif R, Bogokovsky H, Orda R: Diagnosis of carcinoma of the breast by fine needle aspiration cytology. *Surg Gynecol Obstet* 164:506–508, 1987.

15. Keshgegian AA, Kline TS: Immunoperoxidase demonstration of prostatic acid phosphatase in aspiration biopsy cytology (ABC). *Am J Clin Pathol* 82:586–589, 1984.

16. Kline TS: Masquerades of malignancy; a review of 4241 aspirates from the breast. *Acta Cytol* 25:263–266, 1981.

17. Kline TS, Kannan V, Kline IK: Appraisal and cytomorphologic analysis of common carcinomas of the breast. *Diagn Cytopathol* 1:188–193, 1985.

18. Kline TS, Lundy J, Lozowski M: Monoclonal antibody B72.3: An adjunct for evaluation of "suspicious" aspiration biopsy cytology from the breast. *Cancer,* in press.

19. Kline TS, Neal HS: Needle aspiration biopsy: A critical appraisal; eight years and 3,267 specimens later. *JAMA* 239:36–39, 1978.

20. Kline TS, Neal HS: Needle aspiration of the breast—Why bother? *Acta Cytol* 20:324–327, 1976.

21. Kline TS, Neal HS: Needle biopsy; a pilot study. *JAMA* 224:1143–1146, 1973.

22. Kline TS, Neal HS: Role of needle aspiration biopsy in diagnosis of carcinoma of the breast. *Obstet Gynecol* 46:89–92, 1975.

23. Koivuniemi AP: Fine-needle aspiration biopsy of the breast. *Ann Clin Res* 8:272–283, 1976.

24. Lannin DR, Silverman JF, Walker C, Pories WJ: Cost-effectiveness of fine needle biopsy of the breast. *Ann Surg* 203:474–480, 1986.

25. Lundy J, Kline TS, Lozowski M, Chao S: Immunoperoxidase studies by monoclonal antibody B72.3 applied to breast aspirates: Diagnostic considerations. *Diagn Cytopathol* 4:95–98, 1988.

26. Martin HE, Ellis EB: Biopsy by needle puncture and aspiration. *Ann Surg* 92:169–181, 1930.

27. Oertel YC: *Fine Needle Aspiration of the Breast.* Boston, Butterworths, 1987.

28. Palombini L, Fulciniti F, Vetrani A, et al: Fine-needle aspiration biopsies of breast masses; a critical analysis of 1956 cases in 8 years (1976–1984). *Cancer* 61:2273–2277, 1988.

29. Papanicolaou GN, Holmquist DG, Bader GM, Falk EA: Exfoliative cytology of the human mammary gland and its value in the diagnosis of cancer and other diseases of the breast. *Cancer* 11:377–409, 1958.

30. Rosemond GP, Maier WP, Brobyn TJ: Needle aspiration of breast cysts. *Surg Gynecol Obstet* 128:351–354, 1969.

31. Sayago C: Aspiration and surgical biopsy. *Am J Roentgenol* 48:78–80, 1942.

32. Schöndorf H: *Aspiration Cytology of the Breast.* Philadelphia, WB Saunders Co, 1978.

33. Sheikh FA, Tinkoff GH, Kline TS, Neal HS: Final diagnosis by fine-needle aspiration biopsy for definitive operation in breast cancer. *Am J Surg* 154:470–474, 1987.

34. Sickles EA, Klein DL, Goodson W III, Hunt TK: Mammography after needle aspiration of palpable breast masses. *Radiology* 145:395–397, 1983.

35. Söderström N: *Fine Needle Aspiration Biopsy.* New York, Grune & Stratton, 1966.

36. Stewart FW: The diagnosis of tumors by aspiration. *Am J Pathol* 9:801–813, 1933.

37. Young GP, Somers RG, Young I, Kaplan M, Cowan, DF: Experience with a modified fine-needle aspiration biopsy technique in 533 breast cases. *Diagn Cytopathol* 2:91–98, 1986.

38. Zajdela A, De Maublanc MA, Pilleron JP: La fiabilité de l'examen des tumeurs mammaires par cytoponction; expérience de l'Institut Curie. *Chirurgie* 107:193–198, 1981.

39. Zajicek J, Caspersson T, Jakobsson P, et al: Cytologic diagnosis of mammary tumors from aspiration biopsy smears; comparison of cytologic and histologic findings in 2111 lesions and diagnostic use of cytophotometry. *Acta Cytol* 14:370–376, 1970.

2

Clinical and Laboratory Techniques

INTRODUCTION

The techniques employed in our institution are engendered by our philosophy (see Chapter 1). This encompasses the clinician-taken NAB; the use of ubiquitous, inexpensive equipment; the direct smear prepared according to the Papanicolaou method; and screening by the cytotechnologist prior to final interpretation by the pathologist. However, for others, methodology must be governed by particular needs. Therefore, alternatives may be preferable and are discussed.

BIOPSY PROCEDURE

Breast: Palpable Lesions

The tools should be ready prior to performing the biopsy (Table 2.1). The biopsy is an office procedure that augments the clinical findings. It can be performed readily by a clinician who is well acquainted with the technique (Table 2.2).

Disposable syringes and needles are satisfactory and inexpensive equipment (Fig. 2.1). In our experience, adequate samples can be taken with a 3- or 5-cc syringe and 18- to 22-gauge, 30-mm needles; the larger bore is useful for fibrotic breasts or fluid evacuation. For single-hand maneuverability, a syringe no larger than 5 cc is used.[9] For large cysts, a 20-cc syringe may be substituted. The costly syringe-gun is not used by our clinicians.

The patient is positioned supinely, although rarely, small lesions can be palpated only when the patient is upright or the arm is elevated. The skin is cleansed with an alcohol swab, as if for venipuncture. A surface anesthetic agent (1 percent plain lidocaine) is recommended for two reasons: First, it promotes patient comfort, since two to four passes through the skin ensure adequate sampling; second, needle

TABLE 2.1. Tools of Biopsy

Disposable 18- to 22-gauge, 30-mm needle; 25-gauge, 15-mm needle
Syringe, disposable, 3–5 cc
Lidocaine
Slides
Albumin (optional)
Fixative
Alcohol swab

moistening by lidocaine enhances the cellular yield. With the biopsy syringe and an optional 25-gauge needle, a wheal is made by subcutaneous injection of 0.5 cc lidocaine at the periphery of the lesion. Thus, the fluid neither obscures the mass nor dilutes the sample. The remaining lidocaine is totally flushed through the now-substituted 22-gauge needle and discarded, leaving the biopsy needle damp but fluid free.

The lesion is stabilized with one hand. With the other, the needle is inserted through the skin wheal into the mass (Figs. 2.2, 2.3). At that point, negative pressure is applied by continuous suction on the syringe plunger, while the needle is maneuvered back and forth, using fan-like or corkscrew motions. After sample procurement, suction is stopped and the needle is withdrawn. The needle should be localized centrally within small lesions but peripherally within large masses which may contain necrotic cores. The specimen usually is confined to the needle except for cyst evacuation. If blood is observed within the syringe, an additional biopsy should be performed with a fresh lidocaine-moistened needle and syringe.

For direct smear preparation, the specimen is expelled onto a glass slide without needle contamination; therefore, the same needle can be reused for the indicated two or three biopsies. The material can be ejected without needle removal by vigorously pumping the plunger back and forth several times. Another method is to remove the needle, fill the syringe with air, replace the needle, and propel out the specimen. The specimen usually consists of yellow-white or blood-tinged droplets which must be rapidly spread and fixed (see the section on "Specimen Processing" in this chapter).

For fluid specimens, a single pass is usually sufficient. For evacuation of large cysts with the needle in situ, the syringe can be detached with a hemostat and replaced as

TABLE 2.2. Biopsy Procedure

1. Equipment outlay
2. Anesthetic wheal
3. Needle penetration into lesion
4. Negative pressure application
5. Needle maneuvers
6. Negative pressure release
7. Needle removal
8. Specimen ejection
9. Slide preparation

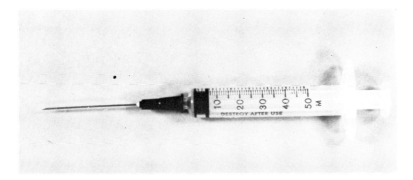

Fig. 2.1. Simple, inexpensive equipment is used. Note the disposable 5-cc syringe and 22-gauge needle.

many times as necessary, or a 20-cc syringe can be used. It is critical to rebiopsy a residual mass (see the section on "Cystic Carcinoma" in Chapter 7).

An alternative biopsy method uses the fine needle alone. The needles are the same, although a 25 gauge needle sometimes is chosen. The specimen is procured by capillary action rather than by aspiration. During needle insertion, the lesion is stabilized with the other hand. Needle maneuvers are vigorously applied within the nodule. After needle withdrawal, a 5-cc, air-filled syringe is attached for specimen expulsion onto the slide. The usual two or three passes are made. This procedure is considered advantageous because it provides reduced tissue trauma, diminished admixture of blood, and enhanced palpatory facility with the bare needle.[4,22] In a study of 632 cases, Zajdela et al.[22] reported that the incidence of unsatisfactory specimens was 5.5 percent compared to 6 percent biopsied with syringe suction.

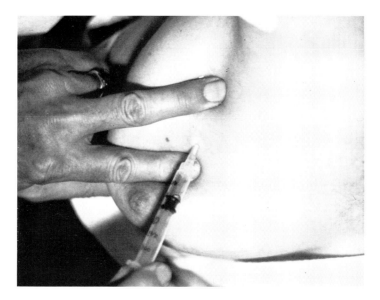

Fig. 2.2. NAB of the breast. Note the needle insertion through the skin wheal and stabilization of the mass with the other hand.

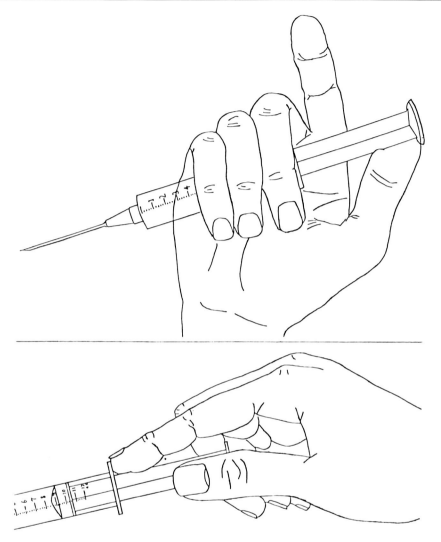

Fig. 2.3. Methods of single-handed NAB. (Japko L: Aspiration biopsy: The pathologist as hands-on consultant. *Diagn Cytopathol* 2:233–235, 1986.)

Breast: Nonpalpable Lesions

Scouting NAB

This simple office procedure provides a preliminary examination of the patient with an abnormal mammogram and no discernible mass. For the procedure, the approximate site for needle insertion is selected by inspection of the mammogram. The needle is inserted in the suspicious region, and the customary needle maneuvers are accomplished over a clock-like frame, with separate biopsy passes at the 12:00, 3:00, 6:00, and 9:00 positions and slides labeled accordingly. Benign cells in this context must be interpreted with extreme caution, although accompanying microcalcifications may make them more meaningful. Superficial lesions provide the greatest reliability, whereas those deeply situated or within a large breast often cannot be aspirated successfully (see Fig. 6.3 and the section on "The Surgeon and NAB" in Chapter 8).

Imaging-directed NAB

See Chapter 10.

Extramammary Lesions

Soft-Tissue Masses

In patients with breast carcinoma, investigation of suspicious, superficial soft-tissue masses by NAB can prove invaluable for staging or diagnosis of metastases (see Chapter 9). The technique is identical to that of NAB of the breast.

Deep tissue masses identified by ultrasonography, computed tomography, or lymphangiography can also be biopsied readily before or after therapy for carcinoma. The NAB generally is performed in the radiology suite; these techniques are addressed in detail elsewhere.[18]

Bone

NAB is a valuable tool for assay of bone lesions in patients with treated or newly discovered breast carcinoma. It can be an office procedure for patients with large osteolytic lesions. For patients with small lesions, those involving the vertebrae, or positive areas demonstrated by bone scan, the needle must be positioned under radiographic guidance. To biopsy osteolytic tumors, a 30-mm (standard), 90-mm (spinal), or 120-mm (Chiba), 22- or 23-gauge needle is employed. It is inserted percutaneously directly into the bone, often at the point of maximal tenderness. To biopsy osteoblastic tumors, a trephine needle (e.g., Jamshidi or Turkell) is needed, followed by the fine needle, which is threaded through its lumen for the customary passes. The biopsy procedure with multiple passes is similar to that used with breast masses, but gentle rotation rather than vigorous needle maneuvers prevents hemodilution. In sizable lesions, biopsy is more successful at the periphery.

SPECIMEN PROCESSING

Direct Slide Preparation

Specimen preparation directly on a slide is the simplest and fastest way of processing aspirates from solid lesions and small cysts (± 0.5 cc). For the Papanicolaou method, slide preparation and fixation must be performed rapidly to prevent drying.

A suitably filmed slide can be prepared in two ways: by the diffuse or the concentrated technique. We use clear glass slides frosted at one end for labeling. For alcohol fixation, albumin-coated or frosted slides are indicated for cellular adherence. When immunochemical procedures may be performed, denatured albumin is used to prevent background staining. For the diffusely spread smear, the specimen is vigorously ejected centrally onto one slide; the second slide is placed over the first, and the two are pulled apart and immediately fixed. Alternatively, a single slide can

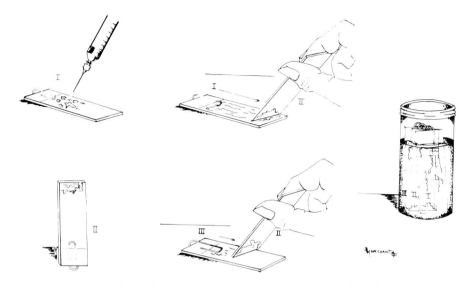

Fig. 2.4. Concentrated thin-film preparation. (Kline TS: *Guides to Clinical Aspiration Biopsy: Prostate.* New York, Igaku-Shoin, 1985, p 13.)

be filmed alone with a wooden applicator. For the concentrated technique, a coverslip or second slide is used as a scraper. The specimen is transferred to the edge of the scraper. Thereafter, by employing the specimen-laden scraper to rub against one or more slides, the concentrated film is made (Fig. 2.4). For bloody or fluid-diluted specimens, prior to scraper transference the original aspirate-containing slide is tilted, permitting the liquid to be filtered off onto gauze or paper toweling.[1]

Fixation, eliminated in the Romanovsky technique, must be immediate for the Papanicolaou method, using either 95 percent ethanol or a commercial spray. The latter is held about 8 inches from the slide for even dispersal over its surface. According to Chan and Kung,[5] cell-distortion from drying artefact can be ameliorated for slides that have been left unfixed for no more than 30 minutes, by a 30-second bath in normal saline prior to staining.

Fluid in small quantities (<0.5 cc) may be prepared as direct smears. For this we use fully frosted, albuminized slides and spray fixation. Larger amounts are processed by centrifugation; the supernatant is discarded and the sediment treated as a direct smear. Membrane filtration and cytospin are alternative methods.

Alternative Preparatory Techniques

Optional preparation methods include membrane filtration, cytocentrifugation (cytospin),[6] and cell block preparation. These provide maximum cell retrieval from specimens taken by relatively unskilled clinicians.

Membrane Filtration

The needle and syringe are rinsed in balanced saline or carbowax solution. The former can be preserved for 24 hours, with refrigeration while the latter can be preserved indefinitely with no refrigeration.

MEMBRANE FILTER TECHNIQUE*

Material

Millipore filters, 19 × 42 mm, pore size 3.0 mm (Millipore Corp.)

Method

1. Moisten the filter in 95 percent alcohol.
2. Place the filter on the moistened (95 percent alcohol) filter holder. Secure on the funnel and clamp.
3. Add a small amount of balanced saline solution to the funnel.
4. Start the vacuum and slowly add the uniform cell suspension until the filtration process slows, using care not to crowd the filter.
5. Fix the cells in situ by adding a few milliliters of 95 percent alcohol. For hemorrhagic specimens, use 70 percent alcohol (for lysis) before 95% alcohol. Stop the vacuum.
6. Remove the membrane and place it, cell side up, in a (Petri) dish containing 95 percent ethanol for fixation for 2 to 10 minutes before staining. (Filters may remain in 95 percent alcohol overnight).
7. Stain by the Papanicolaou method, with the following exception: clear for 1 to 2 minutes with absolute isopropyl alcohol instead of ethyl alcohol.
8. Clear with xylol
9. Mount the specimen.

Cell Block

Paraffin-block sections can be made from clotted specimens or tissue fragments. For specimens collected in carbowax solution, centrifugation provides a button for cell block. This method can also be employed for specimens ejected directly into formalin.[2,3] For pathologists, cell blocks provide architecture similar to that of histologic sections. This, however, is a more costly procedure and necessitates a 24-hour delay for processing.

Stains*

Following specimen fixation, the preparatory process can be interrupted indefinitely. Thereafter, the Papanicolaou or hematoxylin and eosin stains can be applied. For air-dried specimens, the Diff-Quik or May-Grünwald-Giemsa stains are customary. A wide variety of histochemical and immunochemical stains can be applied as indicated.[10]

Generally, decolorization is unnecessary. Most special stains, including immunocytochemical reactions, can be applied to the direct-smear Papanicolaou preparation but not to the membrane filter specimen. After interpretation, many special stains can be decolorized and the Papanicolaou stain reapplied.

---

*Membrane filter technique and all stains: Kline TS: *Handbook of Fine Needle Aspiration Biopsy Cytology,* ed 2. New York, Churchill Livingstone, 1988. Used by permission.

PAPANICOLAOU QUICK STAIN*

Fixation

95 percent alcohol   1 minute

Procedure

Tap water   5–10 dips
Hematoxylin (Gill's)   30–60 seconds
Tap water   10 dips
95 percent alcohol   10 dips
OG-6   30 seconds
95 percent alcohol   5 dips
EA-65   30 seconds
95 percent alcohol   5–10 dips

Absolute alcohol   30 seconds
Xylol   30 seconds (clear)
Mount

HEMOTOXYLIN-EOSIN QUICK STAIN**

Fixation

95 percent alcohol   1 minute

Procedure

Tap water   Clear
Hematoxylin   1 minute
Tap water   Rinse
Eosin   30 seconds
95 percent alcohol   10 dips
Absolute alcohol   10 dips
Xylol   10 dips
Mount

MUCICARMINE STAIN**

Special Solution

Mayer's mucicarmine solution†
Mucicarmine   1 part
Tap water   4 parts

* Source: Sachdeva R, Kline TS: Aspiration biopsy cytology and special stains. *Acta Cytol* 25:678–683, 1981.

**Sources: Sachdeva R, Kline TS: Aspiration biopsy cytology and special stains. *Acta Cytol* 25:678–683, 1981. Sheehan DC, Hrapchak BB: *Theory and Practice of Histotechnology,* ed 2. St. Louis, CV Mosby, 1980.

† Poly Scientific Labs, Bayshore, New York.

Fixation

95 percent alcohol, 10 percent formalin, or air dry

Procedure

Hematoxylin	5 minutes
Tap water	30 seconds
Mayer's mucicarmine solution	30 minutes
Tap water	30 seconds
70 percent alcohol	10 dips
95 percent alcohol	10 dips
Eosin-azure	30 seconds
95 percent alcohol	10 dips
Absolute alcohol	2 minutes
Xylol	4 minutes
Mount	

Results

Mucin: red to magenta

PROCEDURAL CHOICES

The method of biopsy and each step of the processing can be controversial.[11] There is no universal procedure that is correct for all purposes (Table 2.3).

The methodology used in our laboratory is based on almost 20 years of trial-and-error experience. We recommend that the clinician perform the biopsy. Therefore, NAB becomes an integral part of every breast examination. The American Board of Gynecology concurs (see the section on "The Gynecologist and NAB" in Chapter 8). Clinicians then become a vital force in the checks and balances required for final diagnosis. Clinicians[14,15] can perform adequate biopsies when properly motivated and instructed. We suggest the use of the disposable needle and syringe because of their availability and nominal price. We prefer the direct smear method for breast aspirations for reasons of rapidity of preparation and cost effectiveness. In other organs, we employ membrane filtration and cell block preparation whenever indicated.[10] We like ethanol fixation because of its minimal cell distortion. For slides sent to the laboratory, we suggest carbowax or spray fixation. We utilize the Papanicolaou method because of our long experience with it. Staining time can be reduced to less than 5 minutes by the use of the rapid Papanicolaou stain.[16] Speed is essential in our busy laboratory, where the clinician frequently requests an immediate diagnosis.

Alternatives unquestionably are successful. European investigators have promulgated a single person as biopsy performer and interpreter (see the section on "History" in Chapter 1). Advocates of the Romanovsky method correctly contend that air-dried rather than fixed smears are easier for the clinician to prepare. Those favoring carbowax collection[2,20] similarly report consistent results for less dexterous clinicians, but the drawbacks include its higher cost and greater preparation time. Adherents of the May-Grünwald-Giemsa or Diff-Quik stains maintain that background substances such as mucin can be better visualized. Those of us who prefer

TABLE 2.3. Unsatisfactory ABC

Author	Multiple Operators	Syringe Gun	Unsatisfactory
Eisenberg et al.[7]	Yes	No	245/1,874 (13%)
Frable[8]	No	Yes	46/853 (5%)
Kline et al.[12]	Yes	No	135/2,623 (5%)*
Knight et al.[13]	Yes	No	22/881 (2%)
Strawbridge et al.[17]	Yes	Yes	1,205/3,724 (32%)
Wanebo et al.[19]	Yes	Yes	38/398 (10%)
Young et al.[20]	Yes	No	11/533 (2%)
Zajdela et al.[21]	No	No	389/6,400 (6%)
Zajicek et al.[23]	No	Yes	168/2,111 (8%)

*Currently higher because of a recent influx of specimens from multiple gynecologists.

the Papanicolaou stain believe that the diathesis can be equally well identified with experience, and that this stain enhances cytoplasmic and nuclear detail.

INTERPRETATIVE TRAPS

Diagnostic accuracy rests equally on technique and interpretation. Proper technique leads to high sensitivity and specificity. Poor technique is a major cause of diagnostic pitfalls.

Competence in specimen procurement is essential. Two to four separate passes must be routine for adequate sampling unless the ABC is interpreted prior to the patient's departure. Poor slide preparation results in a number of errors. Tumor cells cannot be discerned in the thickly spread smear. Improperly fixed cells simulate cytoplasmic and nuclear abnormalities. Instruction of the clinician in each step of the procedure is the responsibility of the interpreter. Cognizance of these pitfalls, with liberal usage of the term "unsatisfactory," will upgrade the biopsy and lessen these interpretive problems.

REFERENCES

1. Abele JS, Miller TR, King EB, Löwhagen T: Smearing technique for the concentration of particles from fine needle aspiration biopsy. *Diagn Cytopathol* 1:59–65, 1985.

2. Atkinson B: Carbowax fixation of needle aspirates. *Diagn Cytopathol* 2:231–232, 1986.

3. Bono A, Catania S, Azzarelli A, et al: Inclusion cytology by fine needle biopsy in mammary tumors. *Int Surg* 70:119–120, 1985.

4. Briffod M: Cytological diagnosis by fine needle sampling without aspiration. *Cancer* 61:1282–1283, 1988.

5. Chan JKC, Kung ITM: Rehydration of air-dried smears with normal saline; application in fine-needle aspiration cytologic examination. *Am J Clin Pathol* 89:30–34, 1988.

6. Dundas SAC, Sanderson PR, Matta H, Shorthouse AJ: Fine needle aspiration of palpable breast lesions; results obtained with cytocentrifuge preparation of aspirates. *Acta Cytol* 32:202–206, 1988.

7. Eisenberg AJ, Hajdu SI, Wilhelmus J, Melamed MR, Kinne D: Preoperative aspiration cytology of breast tumors. *Acta Cytol* 30:135–146, 1986.

8. Frable WJ: Needle aspiration of the breast. *Cancer* 53:671–676, 1984.

9. Japko L: Aspiration biopsy: The pathologist as hands-on consultant. *Diagn Cytopathol* 2:233–235, 1986.

10. Kline TS: *Handbook of Fine Needle Aspiration Biopsy Cytology*, ed 2. New York, Churchill Livingstone, 1988.

11. Kline TS: The how's of aspiration biopsy. *Diagn Cytopathol* 2:228, 1986.

12. Kline TS, Kannan V, Kline IK: Appraisal and cytomorphologic analysis of common carcinomas of the breast. *Diagn Cytopathol* 1:188–193, 1985.

13. Knight DC, Lowell DM, Heimann A, Dunn E: Aspiration of the breast and nipple discharge cytology. *Surg Gynecol Obstet* 163:415–420, 1986.

14. Koss LG, Woyke S, Olszewski W: *Aspiration Biopsy; Cytologic Interpretation and Histologic Bases*. New York, Igaku-Shoin, 1984.

15. Lee KR, Foster RS, Papillo JL: Fine needle aspiration of the breast; importance of the aspirator. *Acta Cytol* 31:281–284, 1987.

16. Sachdeva R, Kline TS: Aspiration biopsy cytology and special stains. *Acta Cytol* 25:678–683, 1981.

17. Strawbridge HTG, Bassett AA, Foldes I: Role of cytology in management of lesions of the breast. *Surg Gynecol Obstet* 152:1–7, 1981.

18. Teplick SK, Haskin PK: Imaging modalities, in Kline TS: *Handbook of Fine Needle Aspiration Biopsy Cytology*, ed 2. New York, Churchill Livingstone, 1988, pp 17–48.

19. Wanebo HJ, Feldman PS, Wilhelm MC, Covell JL, Binns RL: Fine-needle aspiration cytology in lieu of open biopsy in management of primary breast cancer. *Ann Surg* 199:569–579, 1984.

20. Young GP, Somers RG, Young I, Kaplan M, Cowan DF: Experience with a modified fine-needle aspiration biopsy technique in 533 breast cases. *Diagn Cytopathol* 2:91–98, 1986.

21. Zajdela A, DeMaublanc MA, Pilleron JP: La fiabilité de l'examen des tumeurs mammaires par cytoponction; expérience de l'Institut Curie. *Chirurgie* 107:193–198, 1981.

22. Zajdela A, Zillhardt P, Voillemot N: Cytological diagnosis by fine needle sampling without aspiration. *Cancer* 59:1201–1205, 1987.

23. Zajicek J, Caspersson T, Jakobsson P, et al: Cytologic diagnosis of mammary tumors from aspiration biopsy smears: Comparison of cytologic and histologic findings on 2,111 lesions and diagnostic use of cytophotometry. *Acta Cytol* 14:370–376, 1970.

3

The Breast and Its Development

EMBRYOLOGY AND THE IMMATURE BREAST

The breast begins to evolve by the fifth week of fetal growth.[2] A primitive milk streak, derived from the ectoderm, extends bilaterally along the lateral embryonic trunk from axilla to groin.[10] At the seventh week, a mammary ridge forms in the thoracic area and, simultaneously, the remainder of the milk streak involutes. In faulty regression, supernumerary tissue remains.

By 12 to 14 weeks, the mammary ridge has invaginated into the underlying mesenchyme, and 25 to 50 epithelial buds develop. Mesenchymal cells differentiate into smooth muscle fibers of the nipple and areola. Hair, sebaceous glands, and sweat glands appear simultaneously in the subjacent tissues, but only the sebaceous glands persist. At 20 to 24 weeks, there is increased growth of fat and vascularized connective tissue. The epithelial sprouts become tubules, differentiating into lobular and acinar structures which regress after birth.

During the neonatal period and early childhood, the rudimentary duct system and mammary tissues remain quiescent. There is only slight longitudinal growth and branching of the primary ducts lined by flattened epithelium.

ADOLESCENCE

Estrogen production, activated by follicle-stimulating and luteinizing hormones from the ovary, causes mammary development at puberty. The ducts elongate. There is reduplication of the epithelial lining, with proliferation of the ductules. Lobular buds develop into breast lobules. The volume and elasticity of the periductal connective tissue increase, and mammary vascularization intensifies. Fat is deposited increasingly and functions as a matrix for the growth of the parenchyma. Generalized secretory activity is quiescent until pregnancy.[10]

MATURE FEMALE BREAST

Anatomy and Histology

The mature breast is composed of glandular epithelium suspended in subcutaneous connective tissue and surrounded by abundant adipose tissue.[3] At the surface of the nipple are the orifices of the collecting ducts. These independently branching units drain segmental areas, the lobes, which in turn consist of many lobules.[8] In the resting breast, the scanty epithelium consists of isolated or clustered ducts widely separated by connective tissue and fat.

The nipple is surrounded by the pigmented areola, specialized skin containing melanocytes. Keratinized squamous epithelium, continuous with that of the skin, lines the outer portions of the collecting ducts, and desquamated squamous debris may plug these openings.

From the nipple, the 15 to 20 collecting ducts each lead to a distal lactiferous sinus with folded walls. These serve as expansile milk reservoirs and are lined by a double layer of cuboidal cells. From each sinus are branching segmental ducts which extend into the smaller subsegmental ducts also lined by cuboidal cells.[7]

The smallest ducts are known as "terminal ductal-lobular units (TDLU)."[2] The extralobular terminal ducts open into single lobules, each containing an intralobular terminal duct and its group of blindly ending, branched ductules (acini). Thus, the TDLU consists of a complex containing an extralobular and an intralobular terminal duct and its ductules, surrounded by characteristic loose fibrous connective tissue.[11]

The double-layered ductular epithelium consists of three types of cells: the basilar B cell, the superficial A cell, and the myoepithelial cell. Most common are the cuboidal or low columnar B cells with pale, granular cytoplasm. Interspersed toward the luminal surface are small, dark A cells. The flattened, external myoepithelial cells are discontinuous around the smallest ductules[8] but become more prominent and continuous as the ductal system ascends to the nipple. The myoepithelial cells are surrounded by a continuous basal lamina of collagen fibers and fibroblasts which merge into the loose fibrous connective tissue of the lobule.[9] Macrophages, lymphocytes, and plasma cells are found adjacent to the ducts.

Under the influence of hormonal stimulation, the lobules undergo cyclic alterations.[4,6] In the proliferative phase, the lobules are small; there are few terminal ductules, and the stroma is condensed. After ovulation, progesterone synthesis causes hyperplasia and dilation of terminal ductules, secretion with vacuolization, and mitosis of the basal cells. In the late secretory phase, there is an increase in lymphocytes and, premenstrually, necrosis and sloughing of the ductal epithelium. With menstruation, secretory activity decreases.

The mammary parenchyma is similar to that of the skin from which it develops. Surrounding the individual or grouped ducts are the cellular, fine-textured collagen fibers, akin to the superficial papillary layer. Compressing these lightly stained fibers are larger bundles of coarse, less cellular collagen fibers, the suspensory ligaments of Cooper, akin to the deep reticular layer of the dermis.

The vascular, lymphatic, and nerve plexi of the breast are the same as those of the skin. The intercostal, lateral thoracic, and internal mammary arteries constitute the arterial system, while the veins drain into the axillary and internal mammary vessels. The nerves are derived from the anterior and lateral cutaneous branches of the fourth, fifth, and sixth thoracic nerves. Initial lymphatics arise around the lobules and follow the duct system, progressively enlarging and connecting with the dense subareolar network. The major flow of the lymphatics, particularly from the lateral upper and outer quadrants, is to the axillary lymph nodes. A few drain upward through the pectoral muscles into the subclavicular lymph nodes, and those from the inner quadrants often drain medially to the internal mammary chain in communication with the other breast.[1]

Pregnancy and the Postpartum Period

The breast functions as a secretory gland during pregnancy due to the hormonal interaction of estrogen, progesterone, and other pituitary and placental hormones. The secretory unit is the lobule. When the epithelial cells of the lobule are stimulated by hormones, the cytoplasmic volume increases, and secretory differentiation becomes visible as cytoplasmic lipid droplets within the cytoplasm.

Most growth of the epithelium takes place prior to the third trimester. Thereafter, growth occurs slowly but continuously because of acinar expansion by secretion as well as hypertrophy of myoepithelial cells. Following delivery, full secretory development is reached. The dilated acini are distorted by crowding and partial fusion. The mammary epithelial cells become hypersecretory. Extrusion of the contents of the cells into the lumen plus extracellular fluid produces the milk that is carried by the ducts to the expansile lacteriferous sinuses for storage.[5]

Cessation of lactation leads to regressive changes. The lobules shrink. Most acini involute, although a few persist. Correspondingly, the interlobular connective tissue again becomes dominant.

Senescence

At menopause, the major change is atrophy of epithelial and stromal components. It is more pronounced in the former, and the ductules and alveoli disappear. Because of fat cell proliferation, adipose tissue predominates.[2]

THE MALE BREAST

Breast development in the male is similar to that in the early development of the female. Because of hormonal alteration at puberty, bilateral enlargement occurs in 60 percent to 70 percent of boys. This usually disappears within several years.[10] The adult male breast is a small structure composed primarily of fat and connective tissue interspersed with a few small, cord-like rudimentary ducts.

REFERENCES

1. Ackerman LV, del Regato JA: *Cancer of the Mammary Gland,* ed 4. St Louis, CV Mosby, 1970.
2. Azzopardi JG: *Problems in Breast Pathology.* Philadelphia, WB Saunders Co, 1979.

3. Boyd W: *A Textbook of Pathology,* ed 8. Philadelphia, Lea & Febiger, 1970.

4. Fanger H, Ree HJ: Cyclic changes of human mammary gland epithelium in relation to the menstrual cycle—an ultrastructural study. *Cancer* 34:574–585, 1974.

5. Ferguson DJP, Anderson TJ: A morphological study of the changes which occur during pregnancy in the human breast. *Virchows Pathol Arch Anat* 401:163–175, 1983.

6. Longacre TA, Bartow SA: A correlative morphologic study of human breast and endometrium in the menstrual cycle. *Am J Surg Pathol* 10:382–393, 1986.

7. Osborne MP: Breast development and anatomy. In Harris JR, Hellman S, Henderson IC, Kinne DW (eds), *Breast Diseases.* Philadelphia, JB Lippincott, 1987, pp 1–14.

8. Pitelka DR: The mammary gland, in Weiss L, Greep RO (eds), *Histology,* ed 4. New York, McGraw-Hill, 1977, pp 925–950.

9. Stirling JW, Chander JA: The fine structure of the normal resting terminal ductal-lobular unit of the female breast. *Virchows Arch Pathol Anat* 372:205–226, 1976.

10. Vorherr H: *The Breast: Morphology, Physiology, and Lactation.* New York, Academic Press, 1974.

11. Wellings SR, Jensen HM, Marcum RG: At atlas of subgross pathology of the human breast with special reference to possible precancerous lesions. *J Natl Cancer Inst* 55:231–273, 1975.

4

Fibrocystic Change

INTRODUCTION

Fibrocystic change, also known as "chronic cystic mastitis," "fibroadenosis," "mazo-plasia," "epithelial hyperplasia," "adenofibromatosis," "Schimmelbusch's disease," and "fibrocystic disease," is the most common lesion of the breast, affecting more than 50 percent of women. This designation implies a spectrum of benign alterations ranging from minimal involutional changes to cysts, proliferation of ducts and their epithelium, stromal fibrosis, and papillary tumors.[4] The confusing relationship between fibrocystic change and malignant tumor is addressed separately (see the section on "High Risk Lesions" in Chapter 12). "Fibrocystic disease" has been the usual clinical name applied to this constellation of findings. A recent consensus recommended the use of the term "fibrocystic change" or "condition," with a listing of the specific findings.[7]

Fibrocystic change is associated with a characteristic clinical picture, yet one which may simulate carcinoma. The patient discovers localized, generalized, or bilateral lumpiness, which may vary during the menstrual cycle. There may be pain and tenderness, especially premenstrually.

The age incidence of this condition, between 30 and 50 years, peaking just before the menopause, reflects the hormonal relationship. Alterations are more common in parous than in nulliparous women. In Haagensen's[5] series of 2,511 patients, the age range was from 25 to 77 years, with 2 percent being less than 30. Although most of his patients developed no new lesions after menopause, 9 percent developed their initial lesion after the age of 54. Interestingly, many members of this older group received supplemental estrogen. Estrogen predominance over progesterone is considered causative in the development of fibrocystic changes,[12] stimulating proliferation of the epithelium and stroma.

PATHOLOGY

The characteristic appearance of tissue in fibrocystic change is that of variably sized "blue-domed" cysts interspersed with white, firm, fibrous tissue. Either element may

25

dominate. The cysts vary from 6.0 cm to microscopic proportions and contain clear, yellow, or turbid liquid or inspissated material. The cyst wall is usually smooth and glistening but occasionally shows pink-white, polypoid projections. Microscopically, ductal hyperplasia and sclerosing adenosis with an inflammatory reaction often accompany the cysts. Epithelial proliferation is considered the most significant change because of its possible relationship to carcinoma.

Cystic dilation of the large, medium-sized, and small ducts and lobular acini is very common. The cysts are thin-walled, with flattened epithelium, or else are lined by a single or double layer of cuboidal or columnar cells. They become distended with clear or sanguineous fluid or else desquamated cuboidal cells, foam cells, or necrotic debris. Rupture may occur, with extrusion of debris and cholesterol clefts into the stroma. Cysts of apocrine metaplasia are present in about 67 percent of the cases.[2] These "red" cysts are bordered by oxyphilic cells with granular, eosinophilic cytoplasm and vesicular nuclei (see Fig. 4.6). The uncommon mammary duct ectasia[6] affects the large collecting ducts adjacent to the nipple. These large, dilated ducts, filled with inspissated material, have fibrotic walls with periductal fibrosis. Accompanying all of the cysts is a preponderance of periductal lymphocytes with some macrophages.

Sclerosing adenosis is a discrete proliferation of lobular acini, myoepithelial cells, and connective tissue. The lobular configuration is retained, although the glands may become compressed and distorted by stromal growth. The aggregated, small acini with thickened basal membranes are lined by single- or multilayered cuboidal cells. In one form, microglandular adenosis, the small, rounded glands are filled with colloid-like secretions, and in another, there is an abundance of periglandular hyalinized connective tissue. Sometimes a florid acinar proliferation with scant intervening stroma suggests carcinoma. It is distinguished, however, by the relatively circumscribed, whorled, lobular pattern with normal peripheral glands, seen best under low magnification, and by the absence of mitoses, nuclear atypism, and necrosis.

Fibrosis is invariable, in conjunction with epithelial and cystic alterations. It may dominate the glandular changes or modestly proliferate. Fibrosis, alone or as the overwhelming component, is rare (see the section on "Fibromatosis" in Chapter 5).

Epithelial hyperplasia involves the entire ductal network from the subareolar ducts to the smallest ductules of the terminal duct lobular unit. Both the superficial epithelial cells and the basilar myoepithelial cells participate in the proliferative process, which eventually leads to papillary or solid arrangements. In most cases, even those showing exuberant hyperplasia, cell atypia is minimal. The nuclei are large but usually vesicular, with rare mitoses.

The mildest proliferation produces a multilayering of polarized cuboidal cells which partially occlude the ducts. Small tongues extend into the lumens, occasionally traversing them to form microlumens which vary in size and shape.[1] Papillae with well-defined fibrovascular cores may encroach into the lumens, a condition which, when extensive, is termed "papillomatosis."

Sometimes the proliferating epithelium of the ducts or lobules shows nuclear atypism and mitoses. This overgrowth, believed by some to be a precursor of carcinoma, is referred to as "atypical hyperplasia" (see the section on "Atypical Ductal Hyperplasia" in Chapter 12).

ABC

Introduction

During the past 15 years, the majority of our more than 14,000 aspirates have been from patients with fibrocystic change. Although the first task is to distinguish these specimens from carcinoma, a second and not unimportant one is to ascertain that the cells originate in fibrocystic change rather than a fibroadenoma. Both lesions can present as focal masses, occasionally indistinguishable clinically, and both may yield some similar cells on NAB. Yet, treatment varies, and elective surgery for a fibroadenoma may be performed. Therefore, differentiation between the two entities by ABC is significant.

General Features

The biopsy performer amplifies the clinical examination of the breast by palpation with the fine needle. Its tip may be deflected by fibrotic areas. Masses, originally believed to be solid, vanish upon evacuation of fluid from cysts. Conversely, presumed cysts may yield only scattered droplets.

The aspirate from fibrocystic change reflects the same cellular polyglot as tissue section. While distinction among ductal hyperplasia, sclerosing adenosis, and cystic proliferations is not always possible, the pattern of fibrocystic change is characteristic. The ABC is relatively sparse but polymorphic. There are cohesive groups of distinctly marginated, uniform epithelial cells. Apocrine cells, adipose tissue fragments, and scattered inflammatory cells complete the picture (Fig. 4.1).

The relative paucity of cells in these specimens may be difficult to evaluate, since it may be due not only to stromal proliferation but also to poor technique (see the section on "Biopsy Procedure" in Chapter 2). Several biopsy passes, vigorously performed, are a mandatory part of the NAB procedure. The resistance that the needle encounters as it pierces the abnormal area assists in establishing the diagnosis of fibrosis. Upon evaluation of these factors, we interpret as satisfactory the specimen with 3 to 10 epithelial clusters per slide, often accompanied by adipose tissue (Fig. 4.2).

Cohesive cell groups, representing polymorphic populations from heterogeneous lesions, are scattered over the slide. Most consist of monolayered sheets of uniform cells, but there may be multilayered sheets, acini, or tubules. The uniform cells have a modest cytoplasm and vesicular nuclei, generally with no nucleoli.

Linsk et al.[10] described aspirates from 210 solid lesions. In 82 percent there were few or no epithelial cell groups, and in 14 percent there was modest cellularity; cells were plentiful in only 4 percent of the cases. Apocrine and foam cells were found in 12 percent and 7 percent, respectively. Similarly from our files, 47 percent of 214 biopsy-verified cases were cell poor, 46 percent were relatively cellular, and 7 percent were cell-rich (see the section on "Fibroadenoma" in Chapter 5 for the differential diagnosis).

Ductal Hyperplasia

Ductal epithelium forms cohesive groups. There are large and small monolayered sheets, cell balls, papillary groups, and tissue fragments. The cells are relatively polarized and uniform.

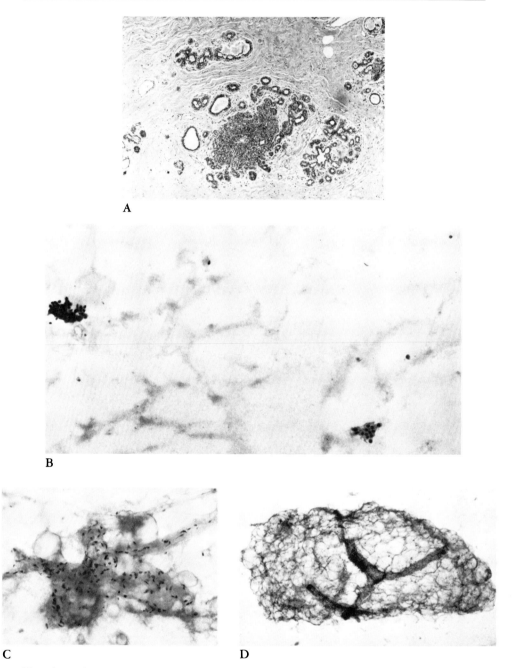

Fig. 4.1. Fibrocystic change. **A.** Tissue section. Note the polymorphic cell pattern with fibrosis. Hematoxylin and eosin preparation (×30). **B.** ABC. Note the sparse, polymorphic aspirate. Papanicolaou preparation (×125). **C.** ABC. Note the mesenchyme. Papanicolaou preparation (×125). **D.** ABC. Note the vascularized fibroadipose tissue. Papanicolaou preparation (×125).

Fig. 4.2. Fibrocystic change, ABC. Note the single group of epithelial cells. This specimen requires evaluation for adequacy. Papanicolaou preparation (×125).

Monolayered sheets of at least 50 cells, sometimes interspersed by lacunae, are most common. Occasionally, there are a few loosely united cells. The relatively plump oval or columnar cells average 15 μm in size. They have homogeneous cytoplasm and vesicular nuclei which occupy 60 to 90 percent of the cell volume and display finely granular chromatin and a few prominent nucleoli (Fig. 4.3).

Other cell arrangements are seen with less frequency. There may be a few cohesive balls consisting of up to 200 small cells and some angulated papillary groups. Rarely, there are large tissue fragments resembling the fronds of fibroadenoma (see the section on "Fibroadenoma" in Chapter 5). A few rounded or bipolar naked nuclei also may be found. In our experience, the combination of tissue fragments and naked nuclei is unusual in fibrocystic change. In a study of 50 of our aspirates, only 16 percent showed occasional large fragments, and twenty-four percent showed a few naked nuclei; by contrast, in 100 percent there were at least three to five monolayered sheets per slide. Nonetheless, the ABC from ductal hyperplasia occasionally may be misinterpreted as fibroadenoma.

Sclerosing Adenosis

These cells generally may be distinguished from those of ductal origin by their multilayered pattern and smaller, slimmer size. They often appear in cohesive groups: multilayered, piled, or in cords which may be interrupted by clefts; sometimes there are a few peripheral myoepithelial cells. Occasionally, small groups are seen. The slender columnar cells average 12 μm in their greatest diameter. The cytoplasm is modest, with centrally situated oval or elongated nuclei. The frequently overlapping nuclei may be hyperchromatic and exhibit slight anisonucleosis (Figs. 4.4, 4.5).

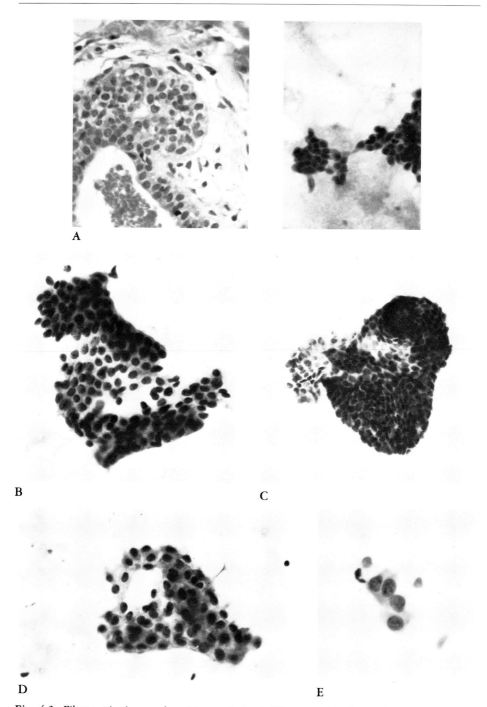

Fig. 4.3. Fibrocystic change, ductal hyperplasia. **A.** Tissue section. Note the hyperchromatic ductal epithelium. Hematoxylin and eosin preparation (×300). **B.** ABC. Note the cohesive sheet. Papanicolaou preparation (×300). **C.** ABC. Note the tissue fragment resembling a frond. Papanicolaou preparation (×300). **D.** ABC. Note the monolayered sheet with lacuna. Papanicolaou preparation (×300). **E.** ABC. Note the loosely cohesive small group of columnar cells. Papanicolaou preparation (×500).

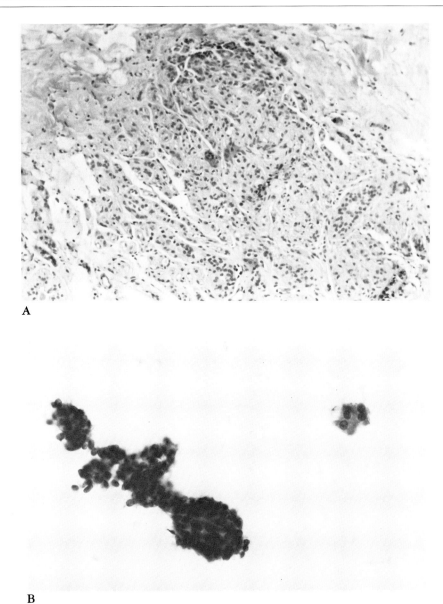

Fig. 4.4. Sclerosing adenosis. **A.** Tissue section. Note the circumscribed, lobular pattern. Hematoxylin and eosin preparation (×125). **B.** ABC. Note the multilayered group of small cells from sclerosing adenosis (lower left), by contrast to the apocrine cells with granular cytoplasm and perinuclear halos (upper right). Papanicolaou preparation (×300).

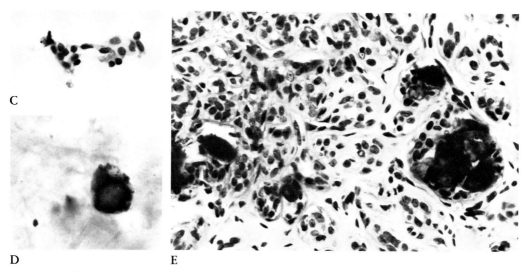

C

D   E

Fig. 4.4. C. ABC. Note the small, loosely adherent group of slender cells. Papanicolaou preparation (×300). **D.** ABC. Note the microcalcification. Papanicolaou preparation (×300). **E.** Tissue section. Note the acinar proliferation with microcalcifications and scant stroma. Hematoxylin and eosin preparation (×300).

Benign Cysts

Introduction

The value of microscopic examination of cyst fluid is controversial because breast carcinoma is rarely associated with cysts. Furthermore, in coexisting lesions, the fluid is generally sanguineous or the cyst partially collapses; in these cases, surgical excision is recommended, regardless of the ABC. But what of malignant cells retrieved from the nonsanguineous, completely collapsed cyst? (See the section on "Cystic Carcinoma" in Chapter 7; and the section on "The Surgeon and NAB" in Chapter 8).

Specimens range from several droplets to more than 30 cc. The fluid is clear or turbid and of varying hues: green, yellow, tan, or brown due to hemolysis. Sometimes it is hemorrhagic, perhaps because of vascular injury from the fine needle.

Cyst contents are minimally to markedly cellular, with a diversity of cell types. Aspirates from apocrine cysts and chronic cystic mastitis may be more cellular than those from duct ectasia. Cells may be garnered from serendipitously sampled solid lesions along the path of the fine needle.

In our laboratory, interpretative terms for fluid samples include cells compatible with "apocrine cyst," "chronic cystic mastitis," "intraductal papilloma," "fibrocystic change," and "abscess." With debris alone, the specimen is termed "consistent with benign cyst contents."

Apocrine Cysts

Green fluid ranging from 3 to 10 cc is generally evacuated from these most common cysts. There is a relatively modest, monomorphic population of apocrine cells in

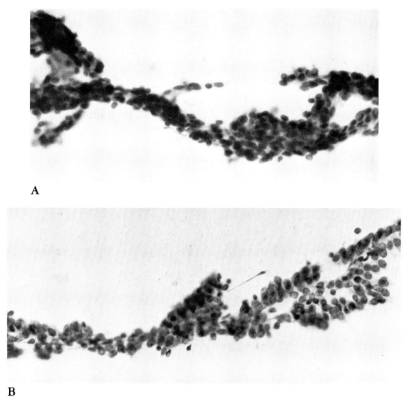

Fig. 4.5. Contrasting sclerosing adenosis and ductal hyperplasia, ABC. A. Sclerosing adenosis. Note the multilayered cord of small cells. Papanicolaou preparation (× 300). B. Ductal hyperplasia. Note the chiefly monolayered cord of larger cells. Papanicolaou preparation (× 300).

monolayered sheets, sometimes interspersed by windows, clusters of up to 20 cells, a few isolated cells, and, rarely, naked nuclei. The oval, polyhedral, or rectangular cells measure 10 to 25 μm in diameter. The abundant granular, acidophilic, or basophilic cytoplasm is distinctly bordered, and the central vesicular nuclei occupy almost half of the cell volume (Fig. 4.6) (see Plate II-2). There may be anisonucleosis, occasional binucleation, prominent nucleoli, or even eosinophilic macronucleoli (see Fig. 4.8). In instances of hypercellularity, the differential diagnosis must include apocrine carcinoma (see the section on "Interpretative Traps" in this chapter; the section on "Apocrine Carcinoma" in Chapter 7; and Figs. 7.2 and 7.3).

Other Cysts

Fluid from chronic cystic mastitis consists of foam cells of uncertain origin. These discrete, large, oval cells, 15 to 30 μm in diameter, display distinctly delineated, pale, granular cytoplasm. The small, round, bland nuclei, about 6 μm in diameter, are either single and centrally situated or multiple and peripheral (Fig. 4.7).

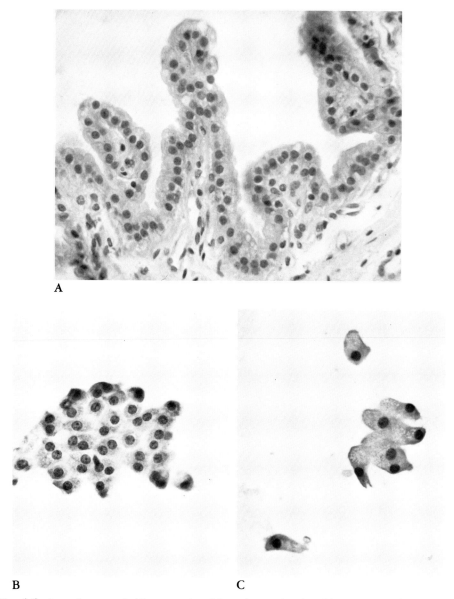

A

B   C

Fig. 4.6. Apocrine cyst. **A.** Tissue section. Note the cyst bordered by cells with abundant cytoplasm and vesicular nuclei. Hematoxylin and eosin preparation (×300). **B.** ABC. Note the monolayered sheet of apocrine cells with cell windows. Papanicolaou preparation (×300). **C.** ABC. Note the oval-shaped and polyhedral loose cells with their distinctly bordered cytoplasm. Papanicolaou preparation (×500).

Other specialized cell groups are linked with specific pathology. Clustered small cells or balls of cells may be from intraductal papillomas (see the section on "Papillomas" in Chapter 5). Innumerable inflammatory cells, histiocytes, and multinucleated giant cells indicate an abscess (see the section on "Mastitis" in Chapter 5). Sometimes there are reactive apocrine cells, large cells with granular cytoplasm,

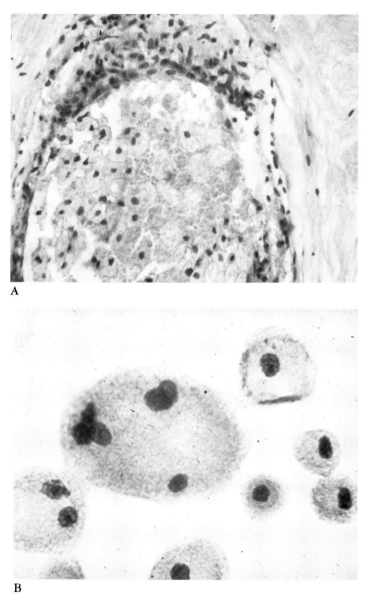

Fig. 4.7. Chronic cystic mastitis. **A.** Tissue section. Note the dilated cyst with foam cells. Hematoxylin and eosin preparation ($\times 300$). **B.** ABC. Note the oval-shaped cells with their distinct granular cytoplasm and small vesicular nuclei. Papanicolaou preparation ($\times 500$).

vesicular nuclei showing marked anisonucleosis, and macronucleoli (see the section on "Interpretative Traps" in this chapter). We utilize the term "fibrocystic change" when a multiplicity of cell types such as ductal, apocrine, foam, and inflammatory cells constitute the ABC. Occasionally, the fluid is cell poor, with debris and a few inflammatory cells. These specimens generally are from fibrous-walled cysts.

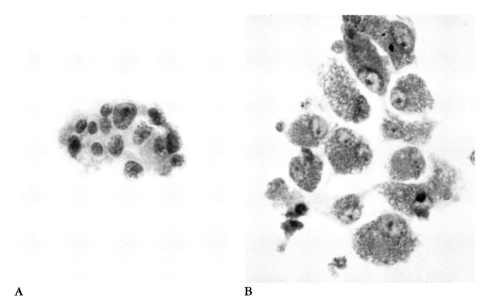

A   **B**

Fig. 4.8. Apocrine metaplasia, ABC. **A.** Note the sheet of cells exhibiting marked anisonucleosis and macronucleoli, but with cell windows. Papanicolaou preparation (× 500). **B.** Reactive apocrine cells. Note the distinctly delineated cells in a cobblestone pattern, with anisonucleosis and prominent nucleoli. Papanicolaou preparation (× 700).

INTERPRETATIVE TRAPS

All large studies include erroneous reports secondary to fibrocystic change. The
incidence varies from 0.1 to 3 percent.[3,10,11,13] In our review of 3,809 benign mammary lesions, over half of the 1.6 percent false-suspicious interpretations were from
fibrocystic change.[8] These mistakes are attributable to (1) apocrine cells, (2) cellularity, and (3) focal atypism. Although most from the first category are avoidable with
experience, those due to cellularity, particularly with focal atypism, require excisional biopsy.

Cells from apocrine metaplasia may exhibit anisonucleosis and eosinophilic macronucleoli (see Fig. 7.3). The reactive apocrine cells appear most subject to diagnostic error, according to our referral practice. Architecturally, these resemble
squamous-type metaplastic cells with molded yet isolated cells in a cobblestone
arrangement (Fig. 4.8). The finding of granular, well-defined cytoplasm and the
absence of necrosis indicate benign disease. In fact, atypical cells with abundant
granular cytoplasm and vesicular nuclei should not be interpreted as positive unless
the specimen shows all the malignant criteria.

Specimens consisting of abundant cells in association with fibrocystic change can
be disturbing. While cell-rich aspirates in conjunction with pregnancy are not unusual (see the section on "Interpretative Traps" in Chapter 5), those from postmenopausal women, the group with a high incidence of carcinoma and a relatively
low incidence of fibrocystic change, are worrisome to us, despite Kramer and
Rush's[9] autopsy study demonstrating intraductal hyperplasia in 69% and adenosis in
57 percent of this age group (Fig. 4.9). In specimens from the ipsilateral or contra-

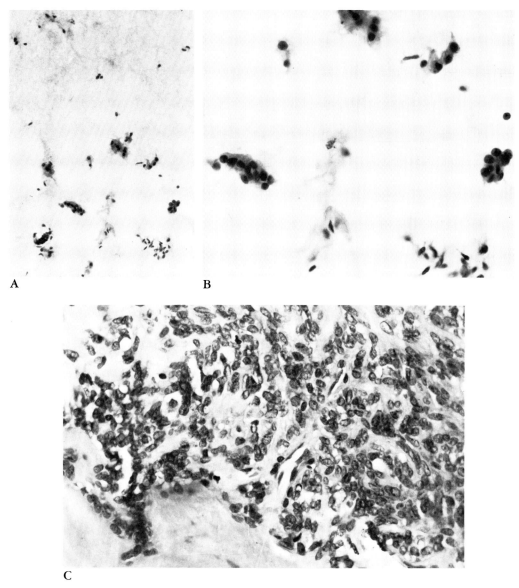

Fig. 4.9. False suspicious interpretation, nodular sclerosing adenosis in a 79-year-old woman. **A.** ABC. Note the cellularity. Papanicolaou preparation (×125). **B.** ABC, higher magnification. Note the polymorphic cells. Papanicolaou preparation (×300). **C.** Tissue section. Note the bland cells. Hematoxylin and eosin preparation (×300).

lateral breast of a woman after therapy for mammary carcinoma, especially the lobular variety, even a modestly cellular aspirate may engender an erroneous diagnosis. For these problem cases we reexamine the ABC, seeking additional signs of malignant tumor, and discuss the findings with the clinician. Inevitably, some of these patients will require excisional biopsy.

In the panorama of fibrocystic change, some aspirates reveal occasional abnormal

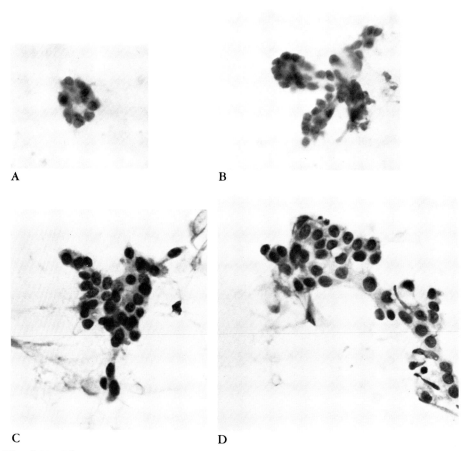

A   B

C   D

Fig. 4.10. False suspicious interpretation, fibrocystic change, ABC. Note the abnormal spatial arrangements. **A,B.** Papanicolaou preparations (×300). **C,D.** Papanicolaou preparations (×500).

spatial arrangements and nuclear alterations. There may be a few cells loosely clustered, in rings, in single file, or in a cribriform pattern. Occasional cells may exhibit anisonucleosis or prominent nucleoli (Fig. 4.10) (also see Fig. 2.2). Carcinomas, particularly in situ and intraductal neoplasms, are found in conjunction with fibrocystic change. The NAB may retrieve only a few malignant cells, whereas the majority are benign (see the section on "High Risk Lesions," Chapter 12). Consequently, these patients usually must undergo excisional biopsy. In the future, monoclonal antibodies such as MAb B72.3 may greatly reduce these errors (see Chapters 8 and 11).

These interpretative traps must be recognized, not only to avoid an excessive number of suspicious reports but also to prevent false-positive diagnoses. A positive interpretation of a breast lesion in a number of institutions, including ours, may lead to therapy rather than excisional biopsy. Therefore, a positive diagnosis must be based on all the criteria of malignancy observed in significant numbers of well-preserved cells, with correlation of the patient's clinical findings.

REFERENCES

1. Cook MG, Rohan TE: The patho-epidemiology of benign proliferative epithelial disorders of the female breast. *J Pathol* 146:1–15, 1985.

2. Foote FW, Stewart FW: Comparative studies of cancerous versus noncancerous breast. *Ann Surg* 121:6–53, 1945.

3. Franzén S, Zajicek J: Aspiration biopsy in diagnosis of palpable lesions of the breast. *Acta Radiol* 7:241–262, 1968.

4. Gompel C, Van Kerkem C: The breast, in Silverberg SG (ed), *Principles and Practice of Surgical Pathology*. New York, John Wiley & Sons, Inc, 1983, pp 245–295.

5. Haagensen CD: *Diseases of the Breast,* ed 3. Philadelphia, WB Saunders Co, 1986.

6. Haagensen CD: Mammary duct-ectasia. *Cancer* 4:749–761, 1951.

7. Hutter RVP, Chairman Consensus Meeting CAP: Is "fibrocystic disease" of the breast precancerous? *Arch Pathol Lab Med* 110:171–173, 1986.

8. Kline TS: Masquerades of malignancy; a review of 4241 aspirates from the breast. *Acta Cytol* 25:263–266, 1981.

9. Kramer WM, Rush BF Jr: Mammary duct proliferation in the elderly; a histopathologic study. *Cancer* 31:130–137, 1979.

10. Linsk JA, Kreuzer G, Zajicek J: Cytologic diagnosis of mammary tumors from aspiration biopsy smears. II. Studies on 210 fibroadenomas and 210 cases of benign dysplasia. *Acta Cytol* 16:130–138, 1972.

11. Schöndörf H: *Aspiration Cytology of the Breast*. Philadelphia, WB Saunders Co, 1978.

12. Vorherr H: Fibrocystic breast disease: Pathophysiology, pathomorphology, clinical picture, and management. *Am J Obstet Gynecol* 154:161–179, 1986.

13. Zajdela A, Ghossein NA, Pilleron JP, Ennuyer A: The value of aspiration cytology in the diagnosis of breast cancer: Experiences at the Fondation Curie. *Cancer* 35:499–506, 1975.

5

Other Benign Lesions

INTRODUCTION

A number of the lesions discussed in the following sections have characteristic cell patterns. In some cases, nonetheless, a definitive diagnosis will be supplanted by a descriptive interpretation, preceded by the sentence "No malignant tumor cells are seen." Furthermore, dominant lesions, particularly in the peri- and postmenopausal ages, often will necessitate excisional biopsy (see Chapter 8). For a guide to all these common and unusual lesions, however, the following sections are pertinent.

FIBROADENOMA

Pathology

The fibroadenoma is the most common benign neoplasm of the female breast.[24] These estrogen-sensitive tumors are found from puberty, have the highest incidence between the ages of 20 and 35, often are present during pregnancy,[46] and are rare after menopause. During pregnancy and lactation, they may develop secretory changes[42] (see Fig. 5.24). Acinar hyperplasia also has been reported in conjunction with contraceptive drug use.[16,21]

These slowly growing neoplasms are usually single, but up to 20% are multiple, either in the same or the contralateral breast. On the average, they measure 2.0 to 3.0 cm in diameter and cause no alterations in the overlying skin. Grossly, they are gray-white, encapsulated nodules which exhibit a whorled pattern with slit-like spaces. Old fibroadenomas may be diffusely hyalinized.

Fibroadenomas arise from both stromal and epithelial tissues, although the mesenchyme predominates. They are subclassed as intracanalicular or pericanalicular. In the former, the rapidly growing stroma compresses the ducts into thin, elongated spaces, while in the latter the stroma grows concentrically around the well-formed, rounded ducts composed of uniform cuboidal cells with a few myoepithelial cells. Fibroblasts constitute the stromal hyperplasia, sometimes with a few

41

benign multinucleated giant cells.[40] Elastic tissue is almost never found, reflecting the lobular derivation of these tumors. Focal mucoid degeneration and calcification are common, while cartilage and bone are rare. Apocrine metaplasia is noted in about 14 percent of the cases, and apocrine cysts may border the neoplasm.[2]

Some rapidly enlarging fibroadenomas are referred to as "giant," "juvenile," or "fetal fibroadenoma." These must be differentiated from the cystosarcoma phyllodes (see the section on "Cystosarcoma Phyllodes" in Chapter 7). The patients are generally young (of 25 patients, a third were below age 15), and the tumors may become as large as 19 cm in diameter.[2] Microscopically, they are more floridly glandular, with greater intraductal papillary hyperplasia and stromal cellularity than the common fibroadenoma (see Fig. 5.4).

Carcinoma associated with fibroadenoma is very rare, occurring in about 0.1% of all cases.[46] In one series, 16 of 26 were in situ or infiltrating lobular carcinomas and 10 were of ductal origin.[36] If the carcinoma is limited to the fibroadenoma, the prognosis is excellent.

ABC

Many of these tumors can be diagnosed by NAB. The firm, rubbery nodule is freely mobile and distinctly demarcated from adjacent breast tissue.

The pattern of these cellular aspirates appears dimorphic, with massed cells and naked nuclei. There are many fronds and sheets, as well as some single cells. The naked nuclei generally are prominent. There may be occasional apocrine cells and multinucleated giant cells (Fig. 5.1).

The most characteristic group is the frond. This may consist of hundreds of tightly clustered cells, often with finger-like projections. There are large and small mono-layered sheets; many are made up of 200 or more adherent cells, while others display fewer than 50 loosely bound cells. Additionally there may be a few isolated, distinctly bordered columnar cells, with vesicular nuclei having finely granular chromatin and prominent nucleoli.

Naked nuclei are often abundant. Many are bipolar and may show anisonucleosis and macronucleoli. A few elongated, spindled nuclei, measuring up to 9 μm, may be seen. Some[34,60] believe that the naked nuclei come from the stroma, while others favor myoepithelial origin. We postulate that the bipolar variety is derived from the epithelium because of its similar morphology, while the spindle type may originate from the stroma (Fig. 5.2).

Foam cells, apocrine cells, and a few multinucleated giant cells are sparsely distributed. In large studies, apocrine cells have been noted in 10 to 75 percent of the specimens and foam cells in 40 to 100 percent.[6,34,53] A few giant cells have been reported in 10 percent of the cases[53] and are more conspicuous during adolescence than in adulthood (Fig. 5.3).

Fig. 5.1. Fibroadenoma. **A.** Tissue section. Note the chiefly intracanalicular variety, with peripheral pericanalicular features. Hematoxylin and eosin preparation (×30). **B.** ABC. Note the dimorphic cellular pattern of the fronds and naked nuclei. Papanicolaou preparation (×125). **C,D.** Note the mono- and multilayered sheets of cells, with finger-like projections and bipolar naked nuclei. Papanicolaou preparations (×300).

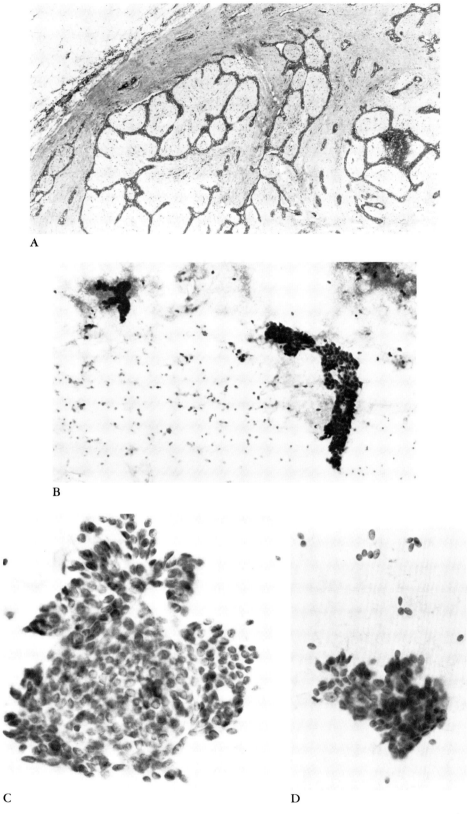

A

B

C   D

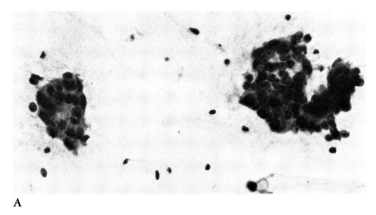

A

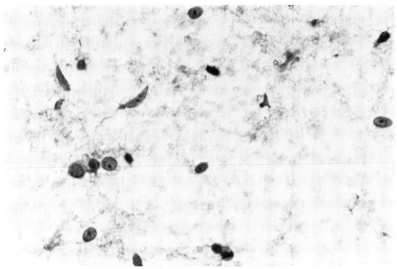

B

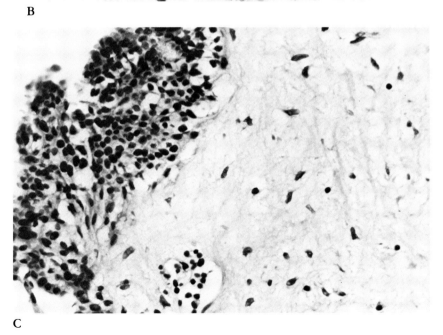

C

44

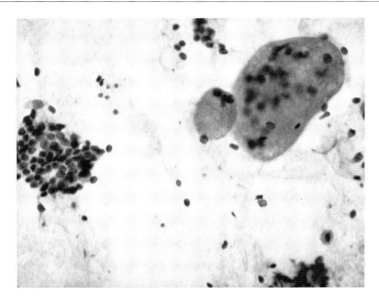

Fig. 5.3. Fibroadenoma from a 17-year-old, ABC. Note the foam and giant cells. Papanicolaou preparation (× 300).

The unusual juvenile fibroadenoma presents a pattern distinct from that of the typical fibroadenoma. There are rare reports in the literature,[12] and we examined a case contributed by Denise Hidvegi, M.D. The cell-rich, almost monomorphic ABC consists of monolayered sheets and papillae composed of several hundred uniform cells. There are also small groups and some isolated cells. Low columnar cells, about 15 µm in length, with oval nuclei displaying mild anisonucleosis and finely granular chromatin, constitute much of the population. Foam cells and histiocytes are also found (Fig. 5.4). The history and the bland cells should prevent a false-suspicious report.

No distinctive groups or individual cells will distinguish the fibroadenoma from fibrocystic change and some of the other benign lesions (see Tables 5.2 and 7.3). Linsk et al.,[34] on inspection of 210 fibroadenomas, noted cellular abundance in 60 percent, stromal fragments in 14 percent, and many naked nuclei in 25 percent, as well as similar cells in fibrocystic change. In a comparable review of 62 fibroadenomas and 42 specimens with fibrocystic change, Bottles et al.[6] described cell richness in 76 percent and antler horn clusters (fronds) in 93 percent of the fibroadenomas, by contrast to 19 percent and 2 percent, respectively, in fibrocystic change. Surprisingly, however, the incidence of naked nuclei was comparable in both lesions. Stroma defined as "clean, clearly demarcated fibrillary clusters of spindle cells" proved the most significant feature of differentiation, being present in 97 percent of the fibroadenomas and in none of the cases of fibrocystic change. We

←——

Fig. 5.2. Fibroadenoma. A. ABC. Note the clustered epithelial cells with naked nuclei. Papanicolaou preparation (× 300). B. ABC. Note the spindle and the oval naked nuclei. Papanicolaou preparation (× 500). C. Tissue section. Hematoxylin and eosin preparation (× 300).

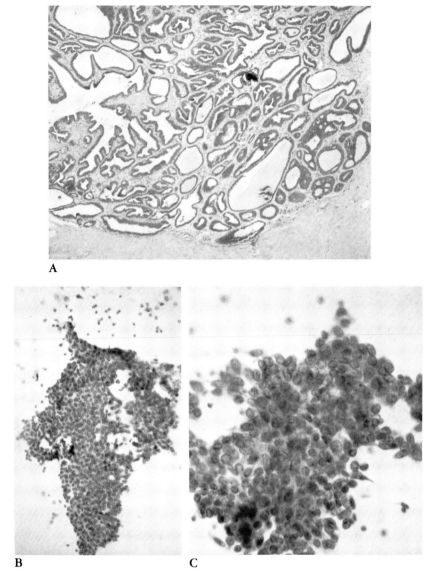

A

B   C

Fig. 5.4. Juvenile fibroadenoma. **A.** Tissue section. Note the circumscribed, floridly glandular nodule. Hematoxylin and eosin preparation ($\times 30$). **B.** ABC. Note the papillated sheet and isolated cells. Papanicolaou preparation ($\times 125$). **C.** ABC. Note the uniform cells comprising the papilla. Papanicolaou preparation ($\times 300$).

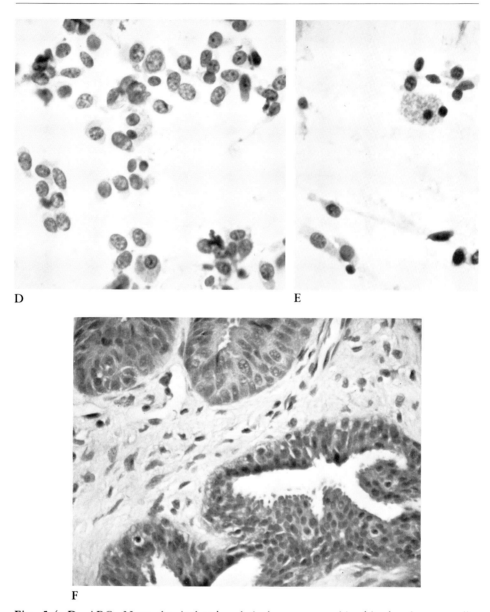

Fig. 5.4. D. ABC. Note the isolated, relatively monomorphic, bland columnar cells. Papanicolaou preparation (×500). E. ABC. Note the foam cell among the isolated columnar cells. Papanicolaou preparation (×500). F. Tissue section. Note the proliferation of glands with bland columnar cells. Hematoxylin and eosin preparation (×300). (Courtesy of Denise Hidvegi, M.D., Northwestern University, Chicago.)

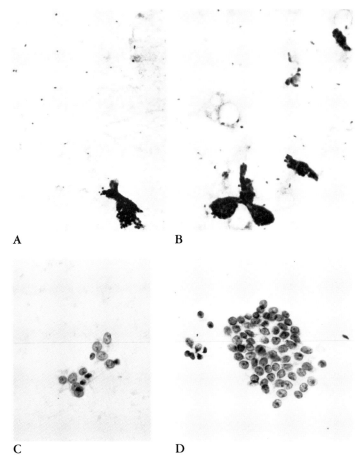

Fig. 5.5. Contrasting fibroadenoma and fibrocystic change, ABC. **A.** Fibrocystic change. **B.** Fibroadenoma. Note the similar patterns, with quantitative rather than qualitative differences. Papanicolaou preparations (×125). **C.** Fibrocystic disease. **D.** Fibroadenoma. Note the similar cells, which are more abundant in the fibroadenoma. Papanicolaou preparations (×300).

were unable to verify these findings in our own material. Utilizing the criteria of cellularity, fronds, and naked nuclei, we identified 65 percent of the 80 fibroadenomas; correspondingly, 7 percent of the 214 cases with fibrocystic change were interpreted as fibroadenoma. We concur with Linsk et al.,[34] who concluded that the cellular findings, leading to interpretation of fibroadenoma in 70 percent of their cases, are quantitative rather than qualitative (Fig. 5.5).

Cells from fibroadenomas have been misinterpreted as suspicious or even positive.[29,55,67] The cell richness, loose cohesion, and isolated cells with anisonucleosis and macronucleoli, common to tumors in young adults and gravid women, are deceptive (Fig. 5.6) (see the section on "Interpretative Traps" in this chapter; Table 5.3 and Figs. 7.10, 7.11, and 7.18). Awareness of these potentially disconcerting findings, smooth nuclear membranes, and the team approach prevent error. Bottles et al.[6] noted atypia in 23 percent and Linsk et al.[34] in 8 percent of these cases, while

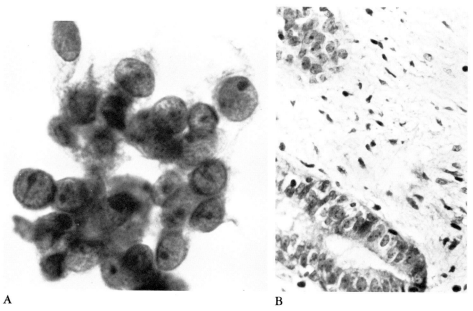

A   B

Fig. 5.6. Fibroadenoma, false-suspicious interpretation. **A.** ABC. Note the loosely abundant cells, with anisonucleosis and macronucleoli. Papanicolaou preparation ($\times 1250$). **B.** Tissue section. Note the similar changes in the ductal cells. Hematoxylin and eosin preparation ($\times 300$).

we[29] reported as suspicious 9 fibroadenomas (0.2 percent) out of 3,809 benign lesions. Currently, our index of suspicion is considerably lower, but it will never reach zero. Rare carcinoma coexists with fibroadenoma, and one case has been documented cytologically in a 48-year-old woman.[54] Therefore, we are particularly cautious in the interpretation of fibroadenomas in peri- and postmenopausal women and request clinical findings prior to the final diagnosis.

GYNECOMASTIA

Pathology

Gynecomastia is defined as "excessive development of the male mammary glands, even to the functional state" (*Dorland's Medical Dictionary*, 27th ed). There may be a diffuse bilateral or unilateral enlargement or a solitary tumor. This relatively common lesion was found in 32 percent of the veterans in a hospital setting[9] and in 55 percent of 100 consecutive male autopsies.[1] From Karsner's[28] classic study of 280 males ranging from 14 to 77 in age, progressive enlargement over a period ranging from weeks to years was noted, with bilaterality in 4 percent and associated pain in 18 percent. Pubertal and hormone-related gynecomastia tends to be bilateral, while idiopathic or drug-induced gynecomastia is usually unilateral.

Microscopically, there are three components: ductal multiplication or ramification; circumductular stromal proliferation; and an inflammatory infiltrate with lym-

TABLE 5.1. Gynecomastia: Cytomorphology of 50 Cases

Cell quantity	
Cell rich:	14%
Moderate:	42%
Cell poor:	44% (<10 groups/slide)
Architecture:	small groups constitute
	50% of the ABC specimen
Tall columnar cells found in 72%	
>50 cells/slide:	11%
Naked nuclei found in 68%	
>50 cells/slide:	24%

phocytes, plasma cells, and neutrophils.[28] Focal squamous metaplasia has been found in about 30% of the cases.[23] In a study of 351 patients, Bannayan and Hadju[4] suggested a time-related spectrum ranging from florid to fibrous. The florid form encompassed maximal proliferation of ductal epithelium and fibroblastic stroma, while the fibrous form consisted of inconspicuous, dilated ducts with minimal ductal proliferation in a dense fibrous stroma. In 60 percent there were occasional lobules and rare acini.

ABC

Although gynecomastia is similar to fibroadenoma, its pattern is distinctive (see Table 5.2). Many times there is a modest cellularity, with variably sized groups of bland cells, tall columnar cells, and naked nuclei. The diathesis is clean, with neither apocrine cells nor multinucleated giant cells. The ABC findings from 50 cases are tabulated in Table 5.1.[48]

There are large, medium, and small epithelial groups. The occasional large tissue fragments of tightly adherent, multilayered cells resemble the fronds of fibroadenoma. Monolayered, polarized sheets consist of about 100 cells. Small groups of up to 35 tightly or loosely arranged cells are most common. Most of these collected cells are uniform, with scant to modest cytoplasm and oval nuclei displaying minimal anisonucleosis, finely granular chromatin, and rare nucleoli.

The bipolar or rounded nuclei, resembling those of fibroadenoma, possess the characteristics of the epithelial nuclei. They average 7.5 μm in diameter and have smooth membranes, finely granular chromatin, and rare nucleoli (Fig. 5.7).

Isolated cells or two or three cells in loose adherence are not unusual. A number of them are tall columnar cells with eccentric, bland nuclei. These cells measure up to 35 μm in length, by contrast to other isolated and clustered low columnar cells, which vary from 15 to 20 μm (Fig. 5.8).

The cellularity of the specimen, with its small groups and isolated epithelial cells showing nuclear variability, may result in misinterpretation. The lesion may be mistaken for ductal or the rare papillary carcinoma because of the tall columnar cells (see the section on "Carcinoma in Men" in Chapter 7). In a series of 43 cases of gynecomastia, 7 were diagnosed as suspicious;[45] we[29] misinterpreted 3 out of 4,962 benign lesions (see Table 5.3).

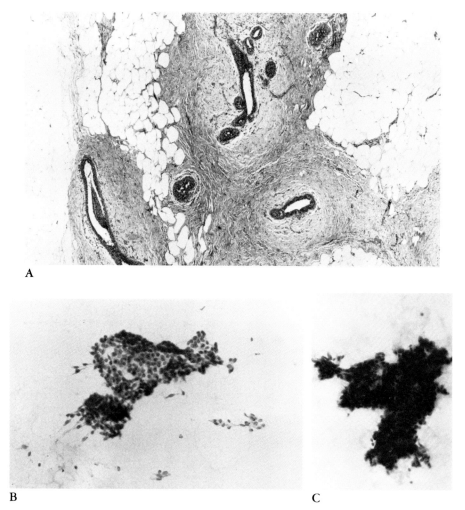

Fig. 5.7. Gynecomastia. **A.** Tissue section. Note the ductal and stromal proliferation. Hematoxylin and eosin preparation (×30). **B,C.** ABC. Note the pattern of moderate cellularity in variably sized groups, tightly and loosely arranged, and some naked nuclei. Papanicolaou preparations (×125).

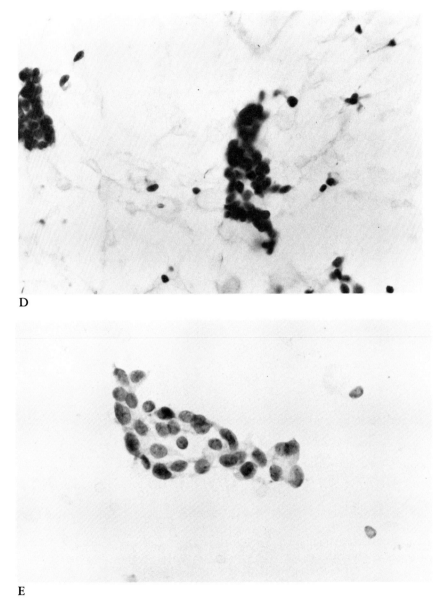

D

E

Fig. 5.7. D. ABC. Note the grouped cells and naked nuclei. Papanicolaou preparation (×300). **E.** ABC. Note the group of loosely arranged, uniform cells. Papanicolaou preparation (×500).

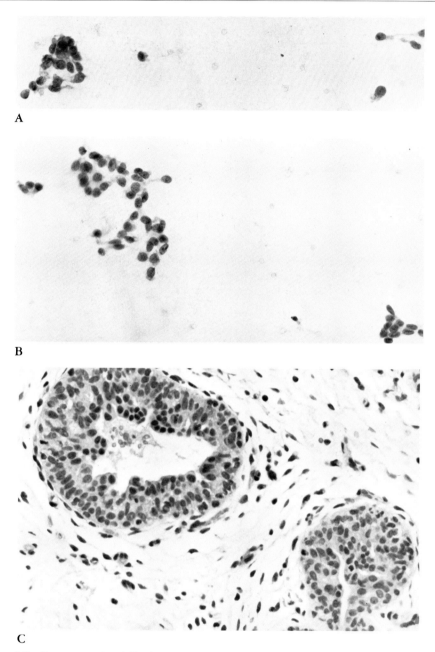

Fig. 5.8. Gynecomastia. **A,B.** ABC. Note the columnar cells. Papanicolaou preparations (×300). **C.** Tissue section. Note the ducts with similar cells. Hematoxylin and eosin preparation (×300).

ADENOMA

Pathology

These unusual tumors constitute 2 percent of all tumors removed as fibroadenomas. The two variants of adenoma, tubular and lactating, probably represent the same biologic process during different physiologic states.[25] The former is found in young, nongravid women and the latter during pregnancy or lactation. Both present as a solitary, well-circumscribed, firm, freely movable mass.

Microscopically, the tubular adenoma consists of closely packed, uniform, small tubules, indistinguishable from normal ductules, within a delicate fibrovascular network. The glands are lined by a single layer of epithelial cells showing prominent nucleoli and some mitoses, and there is an attenuated layer of myoepithelial cells.

The lactating adenoma is composed of large, irregular, foam-filled alveoli separated by inconspicuous fibrovascular septae. The alveoli are rimmed by vacuolated epithelial cells with frequent mitoses and occasional myoepithelial cells, but there is neither necrosis nor atypia. In early pregnancy, the adenoma resembles the tubular type, except that the tubules vary in size and contain oil red O−positive cytoplasmic fat vacuoles.[25]

ABC

Both the tubular adenoma and the lactating adenoma manifest similar cytology. The cell-rich ABC resembles that of a fibroadenoma. It is composed chiefly of loosely grouped and isolated cells and many naked nuclei, as well as a few fronds, monolayered sheets, and cell balls. The cells measure 10 to 20 μm in length, and the often eccentric nuclei range from 7 to 10 μm. The modest cytoplasm is somewhat indistinct and may display occasional vacuoles in the lactating variety, while the vesicular nuclei show anisonucleosis and macronucleoli. The plentiful, rounded or bipolar naked nuclei exhibit like features (Figs. 5.9, 5.10). (See Figs. 5.21 and 5.22 and Table 5.2 for comparative cytomorphology.) The few reported cases[7,17,42] stress the nuclear atypism and macronucleoli (see Fig. 7.18 and Table 5.3). Diagnostic mishaps are avoided by noting the clinical and cytologic similarity of the adenoma to a fibroadenoma, its frequent association with pregnancy, and the youthfulness of the patient.

PAPILLOMA

Pathology

The term "papilloma" refers to a variety of benign lesions with papillary excrescences. These include papillomatosis, associated with fibrocystic change; the solitary

Fig. 5.9. Adenoma. **A.** Tissue section. Note the circumscribed tumor composed of closely packed tubules. Hematoxylin and eosin preparation (×30). **B.** ABC. Note the pattern of loosely grouped cells and naked nuclei. Papanicolaou preparation (×125). **C,D.** ABC. Note the loosely grouped cells and naked nuclei displaying anisonucleosis and macronucleoli. Papanicolaou preparations (×500).

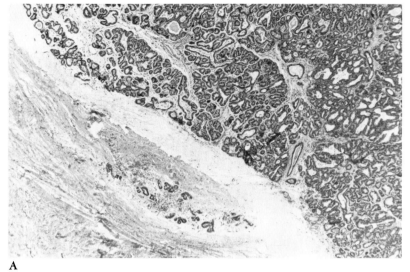

A

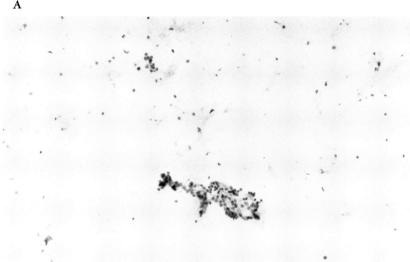

B

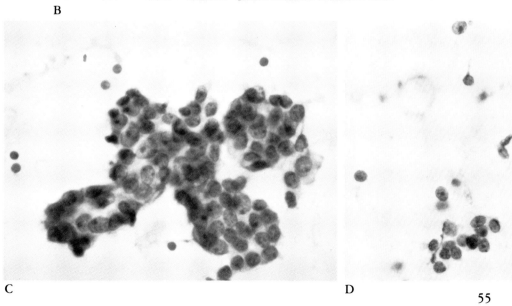

C

D

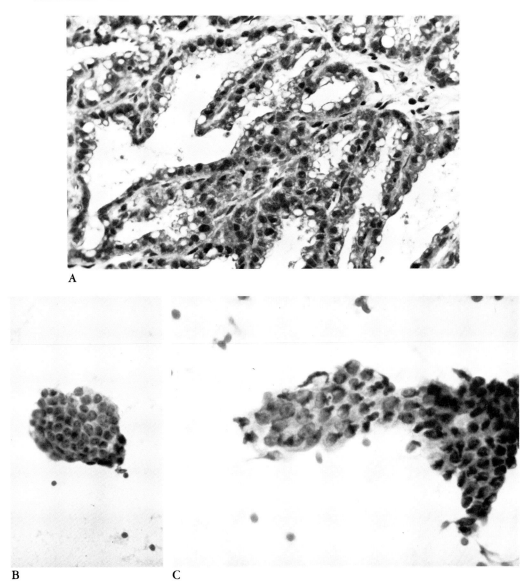

A

B   C

Fig. 5.10. Lactating adenoma. **A.** Tissue section. Note the crowded ducts of vacuolated cells. Hematoxylin and eosin preparation (×300). **B.** ABC. Note the cell ball. Papnicolaou preparation (×300). **C.** ABC. Note the monolayered sheet with cells exhibiting minimal secretion, anisonucleosis, and macronucleoli. Papanicolaou preparation (×500).

intraductal papilloma or papillary adenoma; and subareolar papillomatosis, which is discussed separately. Intraductal papillomas are somewhat unusual tumors occurring at all ages in women and also appearing in men.[50,62] The majority arise in the major lactiferous ducts[32] and commonly cause a serous or bloody nipple discharge. Sometimes there is a palpable, small lump and, occasionally, nipple retraction.

The soft, friable, pink, papillated tumors may occlude the dilated ducts. They may be found within hemorrhagic cysts averaging 2.5 cm in diameter. Some are multiple or extend into neighboring ducts.[32]

The tumors are composed of slender papillary outgrowths with central fibrovascular cores. The ramifying stalks may fill the duct lumina, forming masses intersected by pseudoglandular spaces of varying size and shape. There are two layers of uniform columnar or cuboidal cells, with a few mitoses and inconspicuous basal myoepithelial cells.[49] Rarely, the epithelium consists of oncocytes with eosinophilic, granular cytoplasm.[39] Apocrine metaplasia is frequent in areas of increased cellularity.[32] The delicate vascularized fronds are easily ruptured, leading to occasional hyalinization and thrombosis. Because of possible recurrence, careful follow-up is indicated.[10] For a discussion of the possible association between papilloma and carcinoma, see the section on "Papillary Carcinoma" in Chapter 7 and the pertinent literature.[37,38,43]

ABC

The aspirate ranges from several drops to up to 10 cc of pink, tan, or bloody fluid. Blood-tinged fluid is best examined by membrane filtration and clotted blood by cell block preparation.

The pattern is relatively cell rich in solitary tumors and only modestly cellular in cystic papillomas and those accompanying fibrocystic change. Although polymorphism is characteristic, it is less pronounced in the solitary tumor. Cohesive papillary tissue fragments, monolayered sheets, and papillae are common. Cell balls are found in fluid specimens. A few loosely adherent groups, isolated cells, and bare nuclei are not unusual, particularly from solitary papillomas. Red blood cells and hemosiderin macrophages may constitute the diathesis.

The cells from the papilloma are uniform and cuboidal or columnar in shape, with homogeneous cytoplasm and vesicular nuclei exhibiting finely granular chromatin and conspicuous nucleoli. Occasionally, the cytoplasm displays vacuoles and the nuclei show anisonucleosis and macronucleoli. Apocrine cells may be prominent, and foam cells, histiocytes, and inflammatory cells may be present. In specimens from fibrocystic change, ductal cells are found (Figs. 5.11 to 5.13) (see Chapter 4).

One of our specimens was from an oncocytic-type papilloma. The cellular ABC consisted of large sheets, small groups, and isolated cells with well-defined, eosinophilic or basophilic cytoplasm and eccentric, vesicular nuclei (Fig. 5.14).

The papilloma may be mistaken for fibroadenoma or carcinoma. Although the cellularity, with limited tissue fragments and occasional naked nuclei, may suggest a fibroadenoma, the polymorphism, red blood cells, and cell balls favor the correct interpretation; clinical findings of a periareolar, soft mass and lack of tumor motility are confirmatory (Fig. 5.15) (see Figs. 5.21, 5.22). We and others have misinterpreted cells from both solid and fluid specimens as possible carcinoma.[11,39] Anisonucleosis and macronucleoli may be exaggerated in pregnancy (see the section on "Interpretative Traps" in this chapter). Distinction from carcinoma is based on the lesser degree of cellularity, relative cohesion, and polymorphism of the papilloma, as well as the presence of peripheral myoepithelial cells[30] (see the section on "Papillary Carcinoma" in Chapter 7, Figs. 7.10 and 7.11, and Table 7.3).

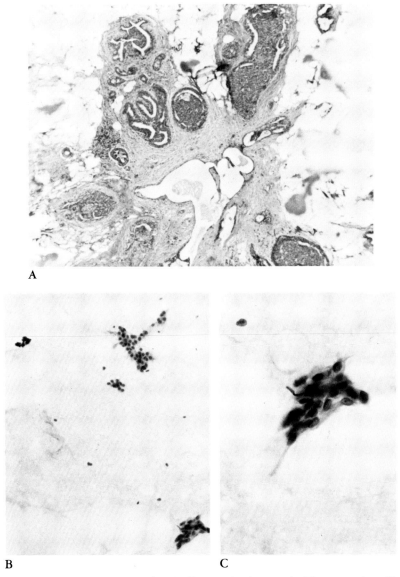

A

B   C

Fig. 5.11. Papillomatosis associated with fibrocystic change. **A.** Tissue section. Note the ducts partially occluded by papillary proliferations. Hematoxylin and eosin preparation (×30). **B.** ABC. Note the pattern of modest cellularity with papillae and polymorphism. Papanicolaou preparation (×125). **C.** ABC, higher magnification. Note the group of tall columnar cells. Papanicolaou preparation (×300).

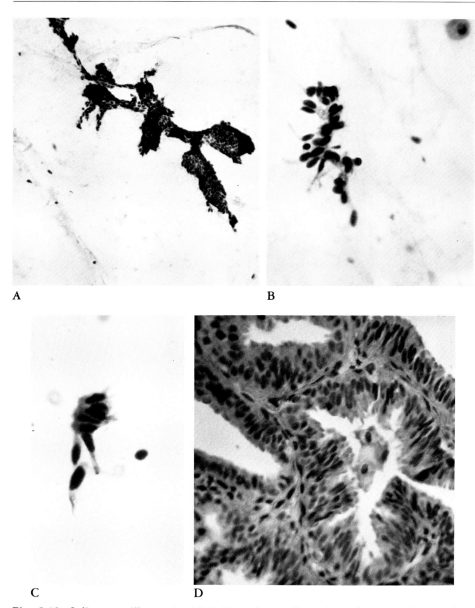

Fig. 5.12. Solitary papilloma. **A.** ABC. Note the papillary tissue fragment. Papanicolaou preparation (×125). **B.** ABC. Note the tall columnar cells with adjacent foam cell. Papanicolaou preparation (×300). **C.** ABC. Note the columnar cells with some anisonucleosis. Papanicolaou preparation (×500). **D.** Tissue section. Note the tall columnar cells. Hematoxylin and eosin preparation (×300).

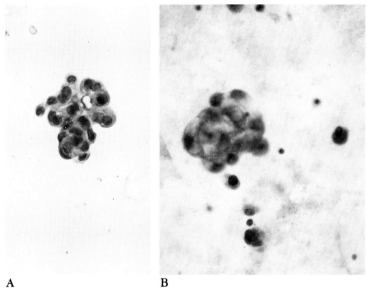

A   B

Fig. 5.13. Intraductal papilloma, fluid, ABC. **A,B.** Note the cell balls of somewhat degenerated cells with occasional vacuoles. Papanicolaou preparations (×300).

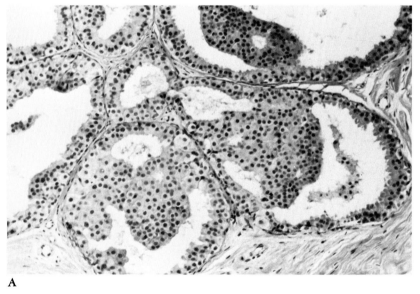

A

Fig. 5.14. Oncocytic papilloma. **A.** Tissue section. Note the ducts filled with papillary groups of oncocytes. Hematoxylin and eosin preparation (×125).

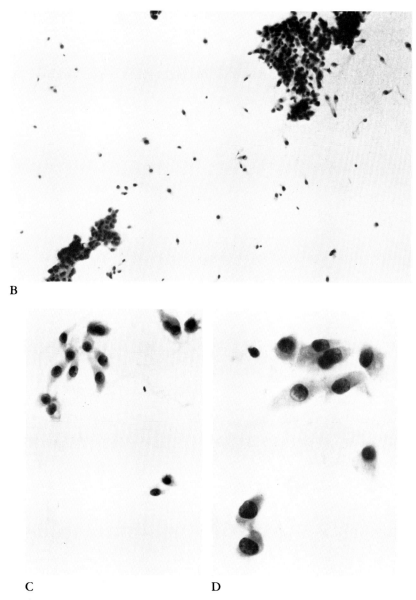

C   D

Fig. 5.14. B. ABC. Note the cellularity with monolayered sheets and isolated cells. Papanicolaou preparation ($\times 125$). **C.D.** ABC. Note the isolated oncocytes with well-defined cytoplasm and eccentric vesicular nuclei. Papanicolaou preparations ($\times 300$, $\times 500$).

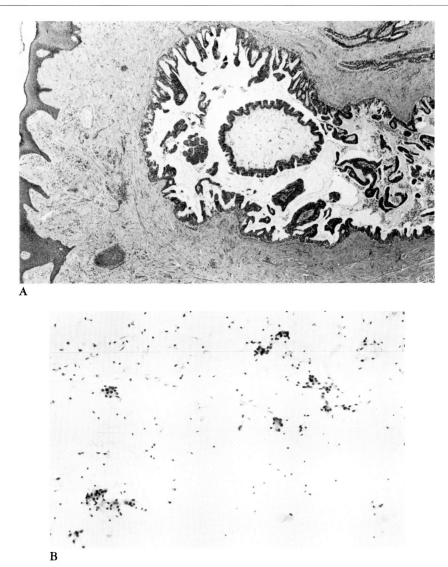

A

B

Fig. 5.15. Solitary papilloma, false-suspicious interpretation. **A.** Tissue section. Note the superficial lesion. Hematoxylin and eosin preparation (×30). **B.** ABC. Note the cellularity with loosely adherent, small groups. Papanicolaou preparation (×125).

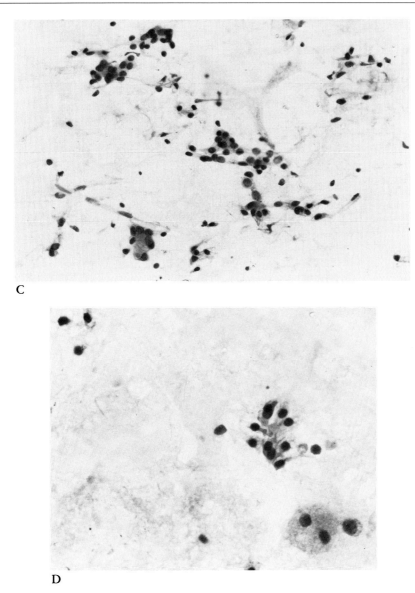

C

D

Fig. 5.15. C. ABC, high power. Note the loosely adherent and isolated cells. Papanicolaou preparation (×300). **D.** ABC. Note the columnar cells with foam cell. Papanicolaou preparation (×500).

SUBAREOLAR PAPILLOMATOSIS

Pathology

This unusual benign lesion, involving the nipple and the subareolar area, is also known as florid papillomatosis" or "nipple adenoma."[27] It is found at all ages, with a mean of 45 years.[44] The ulceration and crusting of the nipple suggest Paget's disease. A sanguineous discharge is common.

The lesion arises in the lactiferous ducts. Both large and small ducts may be occluded by an exuberant growth of branched papillary epithelium with delicate connective tissue cores. The ductal proliferations consist of a double layer of relatively uniform columnar cells with a few mitoses. Myoepithelial cells may be found, as well as nests of apocrine cells. The neoplasm may replace with columnar epithelium the squamous cells of the proximal lactiferous ducts and may expand into the subareolar area, creating keratin-filled cysts. It can be distinguished from intraductal cribriform or papillary carcinoma by the myoepithelial cells and the two-layered columnar cells which Perzin and Lattes[44] observed in all of their 65 cases, as well as by the apocrine metaplasia. It is considered a benign neoplasm, despite reports of a few carcinomas coexisting or developing in the same or the contralateral breast.[47] It must be treated, however, by generous resection because of possible local recurrence.[44]

ABC

The pattern is cell rich, with many isolated cells and naked nuclei. There are also tightly or loosely adherent mono- and multilayered groups. Although the specimen is relatively monomorphic, there are a few epithelial groups of diverse origins.

The majority of cells are columnar, measuring from 15 to 20 μm, with modest, pale, ill-defined cytoplasm. The eccentrically positioned, vesicular nuclei demonstrate smooth membranes, finely granular chromatin, and a few prominent nucleoli. There are many oval, vesicular, or spindled naked nuclei measuring up to 8 μm. Cells of squamous origin form clusters of 6 to 25 cells. Somewhat larger than the columnar cells, they have well-delineated, abundant, waxy cytoplasm and large, vesicular nuclei (Fig. 5.16). Features differentiating this lesion from other benign tumors are presented in Table 5.2 and Figs. 5.21, 5.22).

The squamous cells may be confused with Pagetoid cells but lack macronucleoli, nuclear membrane irregularity, and halos. In one case, Stormby and Bondeson[56] emphasized that to avoid a false-positive diagnosis due to cell density and the presence of numerous isolated cells, there must be close clinical correlation (see Tables 5.3 and 7.3 and Figs. 7.10 and 7.11).

Fig. 5.16. Subareolar papillomatosis. **A.** Tissue section. Note the papillary tumor adjacent to the surface squamous epithelium (lower left). Hematoxylin and eosin preparation (×30). **B.** ABC. Note the cell-rich pattern with many isolated cells, but also some large groups of epithelial cells. Papanicolaou preparation (×125). **C.** ABC. Note the group of squamous cells (upper right) with many columnar cells and naked nuclei. Papanicolaou preparation (×500). **D.** Tissue section. Note the nest of squamous cells (upper right). Hematoxylin and eosin preparation (×300).

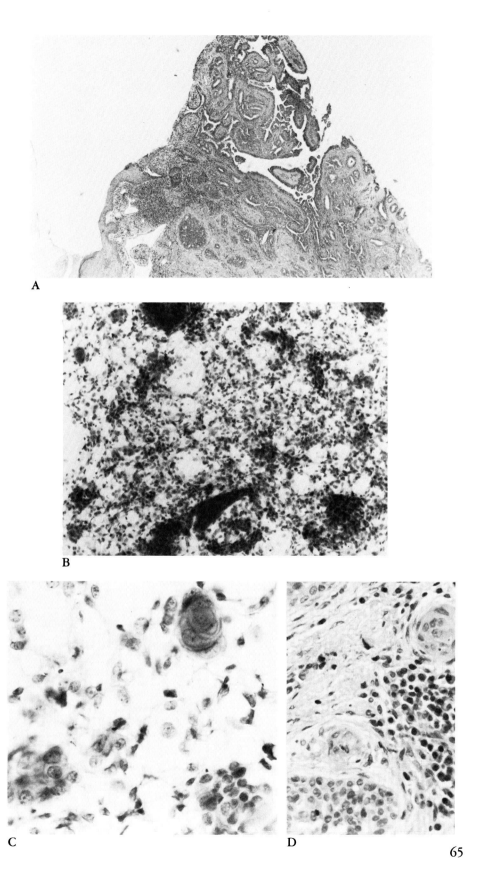

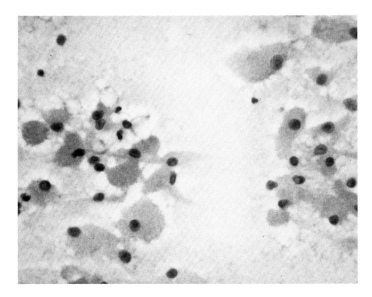

Fig. 5.17. Granular cell tumor, ABC. Note the polygonal and oval cells with ill-defined cytoplasm and small vesicular nuclei. Papanicolaou preparation (×300). (Photograph courtesy of Denise Hidvegi, M.D., Northwestern University, Chicago.)

GRANULAR CELL TUMOR

Pathology

These neoplasms have their histogenesis in neural ectodermal tissue, probably the Schwann cell.[66] Though found in other sites, they are very rare in the breast, having an incidence of about 1 per 1,000 malignant tumors.[22] They are variable in size and very firm. They may show irregular borders and fixation to the adjacent tissue; and they demonstrate a gritty sensation to the needle or knife, simulating carcinoma clinically and on frozen section. Histologically, the diffuse or sometimes encapsulated neoplasm consists of sheets of tumor cells, polygonal or oval in shape, with eosinophilic, granular cytoplasm and small nuclei. The vast majority of these neoplasms are benign, and simple excision is sufficient therapy.

ABC

The ABC is modestly cellular, with sheets or isolated, rounded polygonal, or oval cells. The rather ill-defined cytoplasm is granular and eosinophilic. The small, vesicular, central or eccentric nuclei have finely granular chromatin and occasional prominent nucleoli (Fig. 5.17). The diathesis may be debris filled.[30,58] Positivity to the S-100 protein has been demonstrated.[57] There is one case report of the very rare malignant granular cell tumor in which the pleomorphic neoplastic cells demonstrated all the nuclear features of malignancy.[19]

MASTITIS

Pathology

Acute suppurative mastitis is almost always confined to the early postpartum period, occurring in 1 to 3 percent of all lactating breasts.[64] Staphylococci or, less commonly, streptococci invade through small fissures in the nipple, causing abscess formation. The creamy yellow pus generally is diagnostic (see the section on "Inflammatory Carcinoma" in Chapter 7). Microscopically, the circumscribed necrotic tissue with collections of neutrophils often reveals microorganisms upon Gram stain.

Plasma cell mastitis, a very rare pregnancy-associated lesion, may involve the entire breast. When the inflammation subsides, the residual, localized, firm area simulates carcinoma. The disorder originates in the mammary ducts inferior to the nipple. These become distended with cellular debris and lipid material. Stasis and inspissation result in rupture of the dilated ducts, followed by the formation of foreign body granulomas.[8] Retraction of the nipple is consequent to the fibrosis and scar formation. Plasma cells infiltrate the ducts and interstitial tissue, giving rise to the term "plasma cell mastitis."

Chronic mastitis may evolve from the acute process. Duct ectasia is common. The accompanying periductal inflammation, with an infiltrate of lymphocytes, neutrophils, and plasma cells, leads to elastic fiber destruction and fibrosis.

Granulomatous mastitis is unusual and often caused by specific organisms. Tuberculous mastitis with caseating necrosis and granulomas usually is secondary to tuberculosis elsewhere.[59] Sarcoidosis has been documented.[3] Fungal mastitis may develop from underlying pulmonary lesions. Special stains or culture will demonstrate the specific organism. A rare condition is non-specific granulomatous mastitis. Although its clinical presentation suggests carcinoma, it occurs in younger women and may be related to lactational mastitis. Within the lobules are granulomas composed of epithelioid macrophages, Langhans'-type giant cells, lipoid cells, and neutrophils with varying numbers of lymphocytes, plasma cells, and eosinophils, as well as small microabscesses.[20] Special stains and culture for acid-fast organisms and fungi must be performed to exclude infectious agents.

ABC

Introduction

Clinically, distinction of mastitis from inflammatory carcinoma can be difficult (see the section on "Inflammatory Carcinoma" in Chapter 7). By needle palpation, however, grittiness is lacking, and by ABC the diagnosis usually can be made. Tan, sanguineous, or creamy fluid or a few cloudy droplets are obtained by aspiration biopsy. The former is more common in acute conditions, while the latter is generally associated with chronic mastitis.

The ABC pattern is characteristic. The specimen is cell rich and polymorphic, with some ductal cells and a variety of inflammatory cells and multinucleated giant cells. Occasionally, due to granulation tissue and fibrosis, the cell number is modest

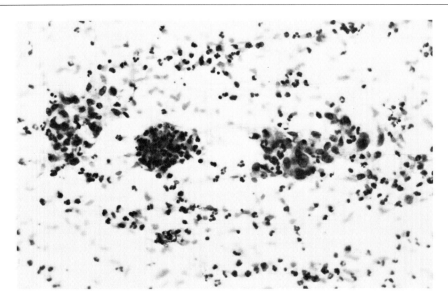

Fig. 5.18. Acute mastitis, ABC. Note the cell density with many neutrophils and dyshesive ductal cells. Papanicolaou preparation (×300).

and the picture is dominated by histiocytes. Because of the cellularity, with loose, small epithelial groups exhibiting nuclear atypism, these specimens may be misinterpreted (see the section on "Interpretative Traps" in this chapter).

Acute Mastitis

The ABC is cell dense, with innumerable neutrophils and debris. Necrotic fat globules are common. There may be a few apocrine and ductal cells in cohesive, polarized units or in small, dissociated groups secondary to edema. The cytoplasm is modest and the oval nuclei, showing anisonucleosis, may have clumped chromatin and prominent nucleoli (Fig. 5.18). For specific diagnosis of subareolar abscess, keratinous material is essential. Silverman et al.[52] noted anucleated squamous cells in all eight of their cases, often accompanied by multinucleated giant cells, parakeratotic and metaplastic squamous cells, keratinized debris, and cholesterol clefts. Three of the aspirates disclosed atypical squamous cells with anisonucleosis and prominent nucleoli.

Chronic Mastitis

The polymorphic ABC specimen may be markedly or modestly cellular. Ductal cells, like those in acute conditions, may be in disarray, with anisonucleosis and prominent nucleoli. Lymphocytes, plasma cells, isolated macrophages, and fibroblasts may be conspicuous or scattered. The macrophages are identified by the well-delineated cytoplasm with granules or vacuoles and by the vesicular or bean-shaped nuclei. The spindled fibroblasts also have well-demarcated cytoplasm and plump, elongated nuclei with finely granular chromatin and prominent nucleoli (Fig. 5.19; see also Fig. 5.23).

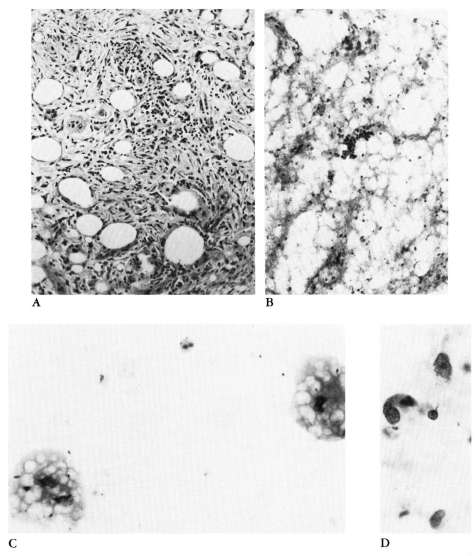

Fig. 5.19. Chronic mastitis. **A.** Tissue section. Note the granulation tissue. Hematoxylin and eosin preparation (×125). **B.** Note the modest cellularity with polymorphism. Papanicolaou preparation (×125). **C.** ABC. Note the globules of necrotic fat. Papanicolaou preparation (×125). **D.** ABC. Note the isolated pleomorphic reactive cells. Papanicolaou preparation (×500).

Granulomatous Mastitis

These aspirates resemble the ABC from chronic mastitis, with inflammatory and reactive cells and a few epithelial cells. Additionally, there may be large epithelioid cells with abundant foamy cytoplasm and vesicular nuclei with finely granular chromatin and nucleoli. The hallmark, however, is the multinucleated giant cell, measuring up to 50 μm in diameter, with central, foreign body type, or peripheral vesicular nuclei (Fig. 5.20).

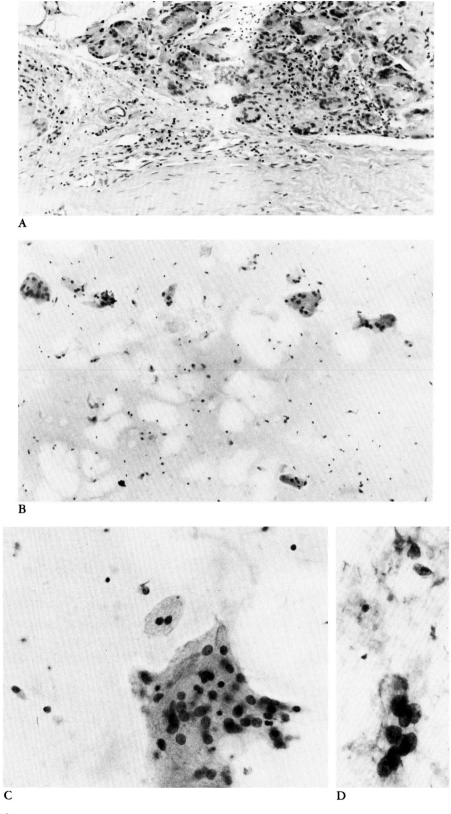

A

B

C

D

70

Causative agents have been identified by ABC. Scolices and hooklets were found in fluid aspirated from a hydatid cyst.[15] In conjunction with tuberculous mastitis, Langhans' giant cells, epithelioid cells, many lymphocytes, calcium granules, and necrotic debris have been noted.[61] In a study of nine cases identified by acid-fast bacilli, all showed a suppurative mastitis, while three demonstrated Langhans' giant cells and five necrotic debris.[26] By contrast, necrosis was lacking in aspirates from sarcoidosis.[5,13]

AMYLOIDOSIS

A localized collection of amyloid, the so-called amyloid tumor, described in a number of sites, occurs very rarely within the breast. Clinically, there is an area of firmness resembling fibrocystic change. Microscopically, it is seen as an eosinophilic, amorphous, nonfibrillar mass, sometimes with peripheral foreign body giant cells. It stains positively with Congo red and displays a greenish hue with polarized light.[35,41]

Several lesions have been aspirated.[33,51] The acellular amyloid resembles colloid. It demonstrates a violet hue by the May-Grünwald-Giemsa stain and is pale pink by the Papanicolaou stain. It reacts to Congo red and polarized light in the manner of a tissue section.

FIBROMATOSIS

Fibromatosis of the breast has an incidence no greater than 0.2 percent. Women, generally in the perimenopausal period, present with a hard mass, sometimes with skin retraction and a suspicious mammogram. On histologic section, there is a dense collection of fibroblasts infiltrating the mammary tissue. The fibroblasts may be multinucleated, with occasional macronucleoli and mitotic figures. In a series of 28 cases there were five recurrences, possibly because of incomplete excision.[63]

Rare aspirated specimens have been reported.[14,18] They have been described as modestly cellular on ABC, with relatively uniform, bland spindle cells.

INTERPRETATIVE TRAPS

Introduction

Cytologic concordance among these benign lesions is not always possible. Differential features are presented in Table 5.2 and Figs. 5.21 and 5.22.

Fig. 5.20. Granulomatous nonspecific mastitis. **A.** Tissue section. Note the granuloma. Hematoxylin and eosin preparation ($\times 125$). **B.** ABC. Note the cellularity with multinucleated giant cells. Papanicolaou preparation ($\times 125$). **C.** ABC. Note the foam cells and multinucleated giant cells. Papanicolaou preparation ($\times 300$). **D.** ABC. Note the epithelioid cells. Papanicolaou preparation ($\times 500$).

TABLE 5.2. Benign Mammary Tumors*: Comparative Cytomorphology

| | Histopathology | | | |
ABC	Fibroadenoma	Gynecomastia	Adenoma	Subareolar Papillomatosis
Cellularity	+2	+1	+2	+3
Fronds	+3	+1	+1	+1
Monolayered sheets	+2	+2	±	+2
Small groups	+1	+3	+3	+2
Isolated cells	±	+1	+1	+3
Naked nuclei	+3	+1	+2	+2
Special features:	Dimorphism	Columnar cells	Vacuolated cells Cell balls	Squamous cells Apocrine cells

*For definitive diagnosis, the team approach is essential.

Sometimes aspirates may be misinterpreted as carcinoma. The pitfalls are presented in the pertinent sections and summarized in Table 5.3. Error also may result from technical difficulties. An unsatisfactory interpretation must be rendered for specimens that have insufficient or poorly preserved cells (see the section on "Interpretative Traps" in Chapter 2). Myoepithelial cells adjacent to suspicious cells have provided an indicator of benignity.[30,65] Upon examination of 3,809 benign lesions, we interpreted as suspicious 57 (1.5 percent): 33 specimens from fibrocystic change as well as 9 fibroadenomas, 3 gynecomastias, 4 papillomas, 3 pregnancy-related lesions, and 5 cases of mastitis.[29] Problems associated with the latter two, as well as skin appendage tumors, deserve special emphasis.

Mastitis

Whether mastitis is the primary process or accompanies a benign lesion, interpretative problems arise. These aspirates must be examined meticulously to differentiate benign atypia from necrotic tumor cells. The problem is intensified in fluid speci-

TABLE 5.3. Benign Lesions*: Interpretative Traps

| | ABC | | | |
Histopathology	Small Groups	Monomorphism	Anisonucleosis	Macronucleoli
Fibroadenoma	+1	−	+2	+1
Gynecomastia	+3	+1	+1	−
Adenoma	+3	+2	+3	+2
Subareolar papillomatosis	+2	+2	+1	−
Mastitis	+1	−	+1	+1

*All may be cell rich. None display nuclear membrane irregularity.

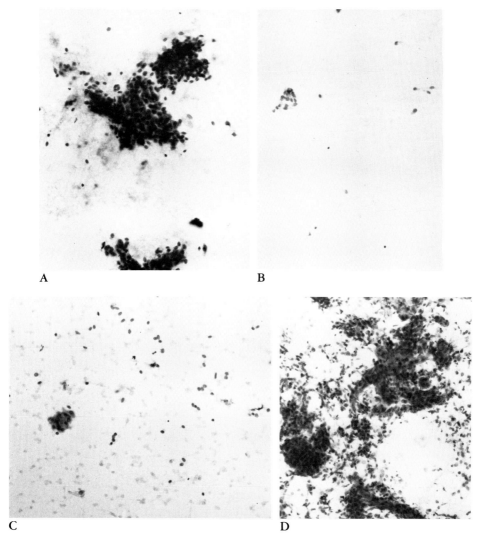

Fig. 5.21. Contrasting patterns, benign lesions, ABC. **A.** Fibroadenoma. Note cellularity with fronds and naked nuclei. Papanicolaou preparation (×125). **B.** Gynecomastia. Note the modest cellularity with small group of cells and a few isolated cells. Papanicolaou preparation (×125). **C.** Adenoma. Note the cellularity with small group of cells and many isolated cells. Papanicolaou preparation (×125). **D.** Subareolar papillomatosis. Note the cell density with isolated cells and cell groups. Papanicolaou preparation (×125).

mens (see the section on "Medullary Carcinoma" in Chapter 6 and the section on "Cystic Carcinoma" in Chapter 7). In solid lesions, too, abundant cellularity, loosely clustered ductal cells, and isolated epithelioid cells, macrophages, and fibroblasts may be misleading. Identification of cells having foamy or granular cytoplasm with smoothly rounded borders and vesicular or bean-shaped nuclei, inflammatory diathesis, and polymorphism help avoid this pitfall (Fig. 5.23). In worrisome specimens exhibiting inflammation, the ABC interpretation of "positive" requires all criteria of malignancy, as well as confirmatory clinical findings.

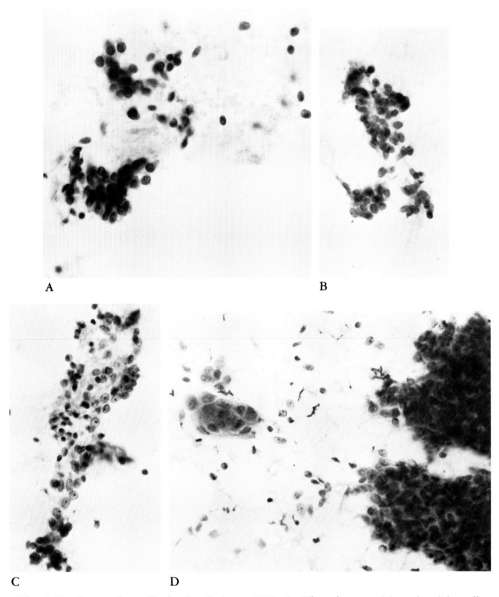

A

B

C

D

Fig. 5.22. Contrasting cells, benign lesions, ABC. **A.** Fibroadenoma. Note the tight cell groups and naked nuclei. Papanicolaou preparation (×300). **B.** Gynecomastia. Note the small groups of cells. Papanicolaou preparation (×300). **C.** Adenoma. Note the loosely grouped cells. Papanicolaou preparation (×300). **D.** Subareolar papillomatosis. Note the squamous cells (left), by contrast to the large cell groups. Papanicolaou preparation (×300).

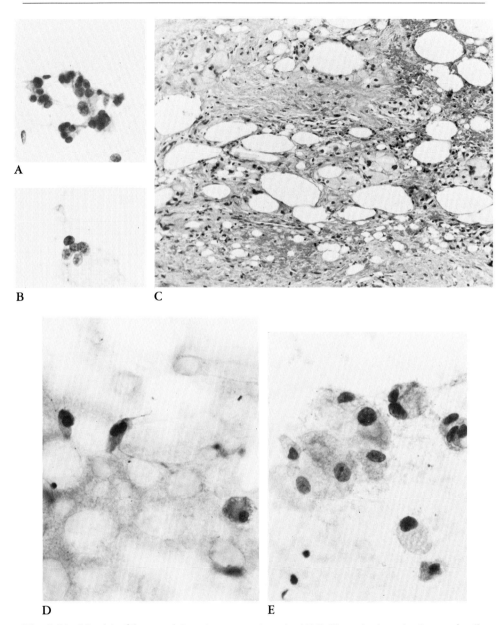

Fig. 5.23. Mastitis, false-suspicious interpretation. **A.** ABC. Note the loosely clustered cells with marked anisonucleosis. Papanicolaou preparation ($\times 300$). **B.** ABC. Note the multinucleated giant cell exhibiting nuclei with anisonucleosis and macronucleoli. Papanicolaou preparation ($\times 300$). **C.** Tissue section. Hematoxylin and eosin preparation ($\times 125$). **D.** ABC. Note the isolated cells. Papanicolaou preparation ($\times 300$). **E.** ABC. Note the epitheloid cells. Papanicolaou preparation ($\times 500$).

Pregnancy and Lactation

Proliferation of the mammary components during pregnancy is a normal physiologic process (see the section on "Pregnancy and the Postpartum Period" in Chapter 3). Similarly at this time, proliferative and benign neoplastic processes exhibit exuberant growth. This results in an ABC pattern that may be cell rich, with diminished intercellular cohesion. The secretory stimulus causes cytoplasmic vacuolization and indistinct borders, while the nuclear changes may include prominent anisonucleosis and eosinophilic macronucleoli. These physiologic alterations, notably in fibrocystic change and the fibroadenoma, have been misinterpreted by us[29] despite the absence of monomorphism and nuclear membrane irregularity (Fig. 5.24). Therefore, during pregnancy and lactation, the diagnosis of carcinoma by ABC should be based on all criteria of malignancy, reflected in a large number of well-preserved cells (see Figs. 6.8, 6.9, and 6.15).

Skin Appendage Tumors

Benign skin appendage tumors in the subcutaneous tissue of the breast may be misidentified clinically and mammographically.[31] They also cause diagnostic problems by ABC. We have examined three such lesions: a ruptured keratinous cyst, a superficial mixed tumor, and a low-grade neurogenic sarcoma.

The 66-year-old woman with the ruptured keratinous cyst presented with a firm mass and a mammogram interpreted as positive. The cell-dense ABC specimen, composed of squamous cells, histiocytes, neutrophils, multinucleated giant cells, and keratinized debris, was correctly interpreted (Fig. 5.25).

The second lesion appeared as a superficial, small, discrete mass in a 56-year-old woman. The cell-rich ABC specimen consisted chiefly of isolated spindle cells with scattered inflammatory cells. The majority of the spindle cells were small, measuring 10 to 15 μm, but a few were as large as 35 μm. All had finely granular nuclei, and a few had prominent nucleoli. The specimen was interpreted as suspicious, and excisional biopsy exposed the benign mixed skin appendage tumor (Fig. 5.26).

The third case was a superficial, firm breast mass in a 60-year-old woman. The modestly cellular ABC specimen revealed loosely adherent groups and larger tissue fragments of tapered cells. The cytoplasm was indistinct, and the nuclei exhibited anisonucleosis, slight irregularity, and hyperchromasia. Verocay bodies with nuclear palisading in a fibrillar substance suggested the correct diagnosis of neurogenic sarcoma (Fig. 5.27).

All of these cases may be misinterpreted if the differential diagnosis does not include a skin appendage tumor. The team approach is requisite. In case 2, the clinical presentation made a malignant tumor unlikely despite the cellularity, isolated cells, relative monomorphism, and anisonucleosis.

Fig. 5.24. Secretory fibroadenoma of pregnancy. **A.** ABC. Note the cell richness with some loosely adherent groups. Papanicolaou preparation (×125). **B.** ABC, higher magnification. Note the small groups of cells showing secretion (right); note the anisonucleosis and prominent nucleoli. Papanicolaou preparation (×500). **C.** Tissue section. Note the secretory cells. Hematoxylin and eosin preparation (×300).

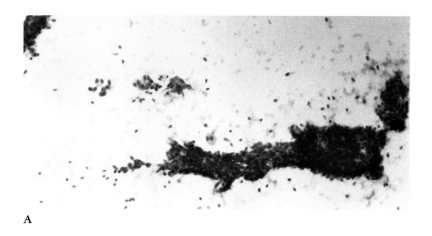

A

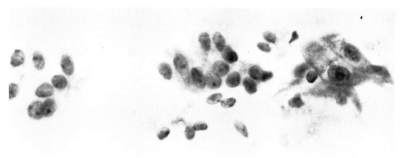

B

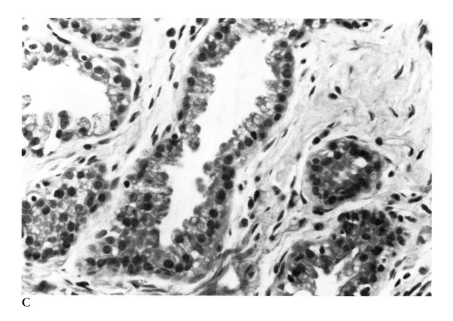

C

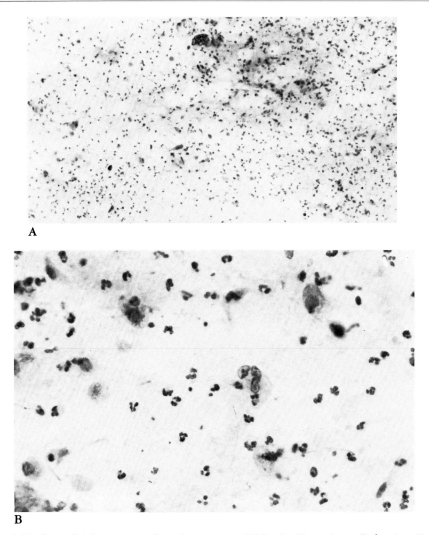

A

B

Fig. 5.25. Superficial mammary keratinous cyst, ABC. **A.** Note the cell density. Papanicolaou preparation (×125). **B.** Note the multinucleated giant cells, reactive cells, and debris. Papanicolaou preparation (×500).

Fig. 5.26. Superficial mammary benign mixed skin appendage tumor. **A.** Tissue section. Note the cellular, circumscribed nodule. Hematoxylin and eosin preparation (×125). **B.** ABC. Note the cellularity consisting of isolated spindle cells. Papanicolaou preparation (×125). **C.** ABC. Note the small and large spindle cell populations with prominent nucleoli but finely granular cytoplasm. Papanicolaou preparation (×500).

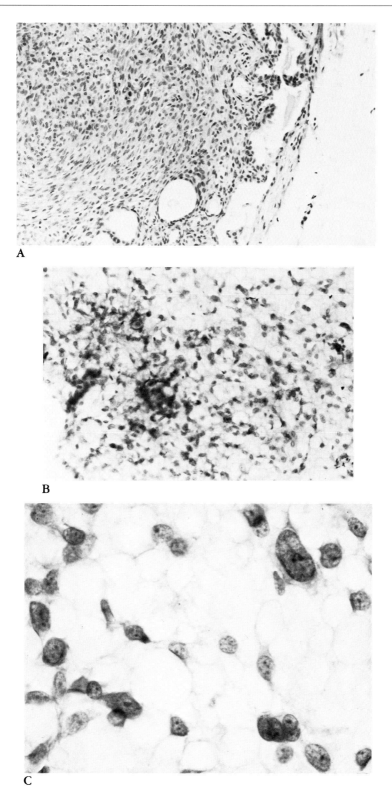

A

B

C

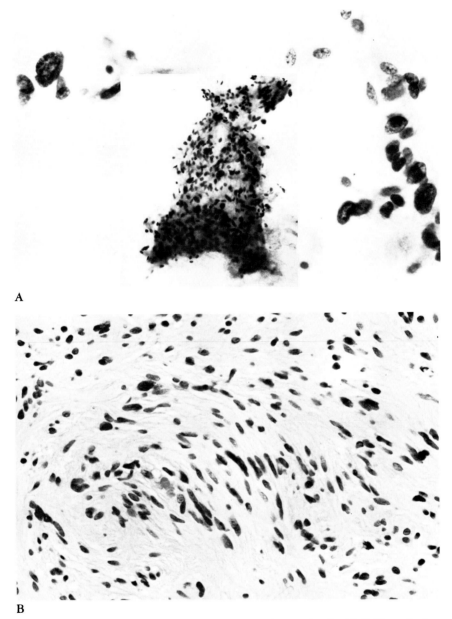

A

B

Fig. 5.27. Superficial mammary neurogenic sarcoma, low grade. **A.** ABC. Note the loosely
adherent elongated cells with pleomorphic nuclei. Papanicolaou preparation (× 500). *Insert:*
ABC. Note the tissue fragments with palisading cells (upper pole). Papanicolaou preparation
(× 125). **B.** Tissue section. Note the palisaded nuclei. Hematoxylin and eosin preparation
(× 300).

REFERENCES

1. Andersen JA, Gram JB: Male breast at autopsy. *Acta Pathol Microbiol Immunol Scand* [A]90:191–197, 1982.

2. Azzopardi JG: *Problems in Breast Pathology*. Philadelphia, WB Saunders Co, 1979.

3. Banik S, Bishop PW, Ormerod LP, O'Brien TEB: Sarcoidosis of the breast. *J Clin Pathol* 39:446–448, 1986.

4. Bannayan GA, Hajdu SI: Gynecomastia: Clinicopathologic study of 351 cases. *Am J Clin Pathol* 57:431–437, 1972.

5. Bodó M, Döbrössy L, Sugár J: Boeck's sarcoidosis of the breast: Cytologic findings with aspiration biopsy cytology; a case clinically mimicking carcinoma. *Acta Cytol* 22:1–2, 1978.

6. Bottles K, Chan JS, Holly EA, Chiu S-H, Miller TR: Cytologic criteria for fibroadenoma. *Am J Clin Pathol* 89:707–713, 1988.

7. Bottles K, Taylor RN: Diagnosis of breast masses in pregnant and lactating women by aspiration cytology. *Obstet Gynecol* 66:76S–78S, 1985.

8. Boyd W: *A Textbook of Pathology*. Philadelphia, Lea & Febiger, 1970.

9. Carlson HE: Gynecomastia. *N Engl J Med* 303:795–799, 1980.

10. Carter D: Intraductal papillary tumors of the breast; a study of 78 cases. *Cancer* 39:1689–1692, 1977.

11. Ciatto S, Cariaggi P, Bulgaresi P: The value of routine cytologic examination of breast cyst fluids. *Acta Cytol* 31:301–304, 1987.

12. Degrell I: Histological and needle-biopsy studies of juvenile mastopathy. *Acta Morphol Acad Sci Hung* 29:365–376, 1981.

13. Doria MI, Tani EM, Skoog L: Sarcoidosis presenting initially as a breast mass: Detection by fine needle aspiration biopsy. *Acta Cytol*31:378–379, 1987.

14. El-Naggar A, Abdul-Karim FW, Marshalleck JJ, Sorensen K: Fine-needle aspiration of fibromatosis of the breast. *Diagn Cytopathol* 3:320–322, 1987.

15. Epstein NA: Hydatid cyst of the breast: Diagnosis using cytological techniques. *Acta Cytol* 13:420–421, 1969.

16. Fechner R: Fibroadenomas in patients receiving oral contraceptives: A clinical and pathologic study. *Am J Clin Pathol* 53:857–864, 1970.

17. Finley JL, Silverman JF, Lannin DR: Fine needle aspiration cytology of lactating adenoma (abstract). *Acta Cytol* 31:667, 1987.

18. Fritsches HG, Muller EA: Pseudosarcomatous fasciitis of the breast; cytologic and histologic features. *Acta Cytol* 27:73–75, 1983.

19. Geisinger KR, Kawamoto EH, Marshall EB, Ahl ET, Cooper MR: Aspiration and exfoliative cytology, including ultra-structure of a malignant granular-cell tumor. *Acta Cytol* 29:593–597, 1985.

20. Going JJ, Anderson TJ, Wilkinson S, Chetty U: Granulomatous lobular mastitis. *J Clin Pathol* 40:535–540, 1987.

21. Goldenberg VE, Wiegenstein L, Mottet K: Florid breast fibroadenomas in patients taking hormonal oral contraceptives. *Am J Clin Pathol* 49:52–59, 1968.

22. Gordon AB, Fisher C, Palmer B, Greening WP: Granular cell tumours of the breast. *Br J Surg Oncol* 11:269–273, 1985.

23. Gottfried MR: Extensive squamous metaplasia in gynecomastia. *Arch Pathol Lab Med* 110:971–973, 1986.

24. Hagensen CC: *Disease of the Breast,* ed 3. Philadelphia, WB Saunders Co, 1986.

25. Hertel BF, Zaloudek C, Kempson RI: Breast adenomas. *Cancer* 37:2891–2905, 1976.

26. Jayaram G: Cytomorphology of tuberculous mastitis: A report of nine cases with fine needle aspiration biopsy. *Acta Cytol* 29:974–978, 1985.

27. Jones DB: Florid papillomatosis of the nipple ducts. *Cancer* 8:315–319, 1955.

28. Karsner HT: Gynecomastia. *Am J Pathol* 22:235–315, 1946.

29. Kline TS: Masquerades of malignancy; a review of 4241 aspirates from the breast. *Acta Cytol* 25:263–266, 1981.

30. Koss LG, Woyke S, Olszewski W: *Aspiration Biopsy: Cytologic Interpretation and Histologic Bases.* New York, Igaku-Shoin, 1984.

31. Kowand LM, Verhulst LA, Copeland CM, Bose B: Epidermal cyst of the breast. *Can Med Assoc J* 131:217–219, 1984.

32. Kraus FT, Neubecker RD: The differential diagnosis of papillary tumors of the breast. *Cancer* 15:444–455, 1962.

33. Lew W, Seymour AE: Primary amyloid tumor of the breast; case report and literature review. *Acta Cytol* 29:7–11, 1985.

34. Linsk JA, Kreuzer G, Zajicek J: Cytologic diagnosis of mammary tumors from aspiration biopsy smears. II. Studies on 210 fibroadenomas and 210 cases of benign dysplasia. *Acta Cytol* 16:130–138, 1972.

35. Lipper S, Kahn LB: Amyloid tumor; a clinicopathologic study of four cases. *Am J Surg Pathol* 2:141–145, 1978.

36. McDivitt RW, Stewart FW, Farrow JH: Breast carcinoma arising in solitary fibro-adenomas. *Surg Gynecol Obstet* 125:572–576, 1967.

37. Murad TM, Contesso G, Mouriesse H: Papillary tumors of large lactiferous ducts. *Cancer* 48:122–133, 1981.

38. Murad TM, Swaid S, Pritchett P: Malignant and benign papillary lesions of the breast. *Hum Pathol* 8:379–390, 1977.

39. Nielsen BB: Oncocytic breast papilloma. *Virchows Arch Pathol Anat* 393:345–351, 1981.

40. Nielsen BB, Ladefoged C: Fibroadenoma of the female breast with multinucleated giant cells. *Pathol Res Pract* 180:721–724, 1985.

41. O'Connor CR, Rubinow A, Cohen AS: Primary (AL) amyloidosis as a cause of breast masses. *Am J Med* 77:981–986, 1984.

42. O'Hara MF, Page DL: Adenomas of the breast and ectopic breast under lactational influences. *Hum Pathol* 16:707–712, 1985.

43. Ohuchi N, Abe R, Kasai M: Possible cancerous change of intraductal papillomas of the breast; a 3-D reconstruction study of 25 cases. *Cancer* 54:605–611, 1984.

44. Perzin KH, Lattes R: Papillary adenoma of the nipple (florid papillomatosis, adenoma, adenomatosis); a clinicopathologic study. *Cancer* 29:996–1009, 1972.

45. Rone R, Ramzy I, Northcutt A: Gynecomastia: Cytologic features and diagnostic pitfalls in aspiration biopsy (abstract). *Acta Cytol* 30:589, 1986.

46. Rosai J: *Ackerman's Surgical Pathology,* ed 6. St Louis, CV Mosby Co, 1981.

47. Rosen PP, Caicco JA: Florid papillomatosis of the nipple: A study of 51 patients including nine with mammary carcinoma. *Am J Surg Pathol* 10:87–101, 1986.

48. Russin VL, Lachowicz C, Kline TS: Male breast lesions: Gynecomastia and its distinction from carcinoma by aspiration biopsy cytology (ABC). *Diagn Cytopathol* in press.

49. Saphir O, Parker ML: Intracystic papilloma of the breast. *Am J Pathol* 16:189–210, 1940.

50. Sara SS, Gottfried MR: Benign papilloma of the male breast following chronic phenothiazine therapy. *Am J Clin Pathol* 87:649–650, 1979.

51. Silverman JF, Dabbs DJ, Norris HT, et al: Localized primary (AL) amyloid tumor of the breast; cytologic, histologic, immunocytochemical and ultrastructural observations. *Am J Surg Pathol* 10:539–545, 1986.

52. Silverman JF, Lannin DR, Unverferth M, Norris HT: Fine needle aspiration cytology of subareolar abscess of the breast; spectrum of cytomorphologic findings and potential diagnostic pitfalls. *Acta Cytol* 30:413–419, 1986.

53. Simi U, Moretti D, Iacconi P, et al: Fine needle aspiration cytopathology of phyllodes tumor; differential diagnosis with fibroadenoma. *Acta Cytol* 32:63–66, 1988.

54. Simpson RHW, James KA, Holdstock JB, Kelly RM, Yankin DHT: Carcinoma in a breast fibroadenoma. *Acta Cytol* 31:313–316, 1987.

55. Stavic GD, Tevcev DT, Kaftandijlev DR, Novak JJ: Aspiration biopsy cytologic method in diagnosis of breast lesions: A critical review of 250 cases. *Acta Cytol* 17:188–190, 1973.

56. Stormby N, Bondeson L: Adenoma of the nipple; an unusual diagnosis in aspiration cytology. *Acta Cytol* 28:729–732, 1984.

57. Strobel SL, Shah NT, Lucas JG, Tuttle SE: Granular-cell tumor of the breast; a cytologic, immunohistochemical and ultrastructural study of two cases. *Acta Cytol* 29:598–601, 1985.

58. Sussman EB, Hajdu SI, Gray GF: Granular cell myoblastoma of the breast. *Am J Surg* 126:669–670, 1973.

59. Symmers W SC: Tuberculosis of the breast. *Br Med J* 289:48–49, 1984.

60. Tsuchiya S, Maruyama Y, Koike Y, et al: Cytologic characteristics and origin of naked nuclei in breast aspirate smears. *Acta Cytol* 31:285–290, 1987.

61. Vassilakos P: Tuberculosis of the breast: Cytologic findings with fine-needle aspiration; a case clinically and radiologically mimicking carcinoma. *Acta Cytol* 17:160–165, 1973.

62. Waldo ED, Sidhu GS, Hu AW: Florid papillomatosis of male nipple after diethylstilbestrol therapy. *Arch Pathol* 99:364–366, 1975.

63. Wargotz ES, Norris HJ, Austin RM, Enzinger FM: Fibromatosis of the breast; a clinical and pathological study of 28 cases. *Am J Surg Pathol* 11:38–45, 1987.

64. Weiss RL, Matsen JM: Group B streptococcal breast abscess. *Arch Pathol Lab Med* 111:74–75, 1987.

65. Whitlatch SP, Panke TW: Myoepithelial cells in needle aspirations of two cases of unusual breast lesions: An aid in differential diagnosis. *Diagn Cytopathol* 2:78–79, 1987.

66. Willen R, Willen H, Balldin G, Albrechtsson U: Granular cell tumour of the mammary gland simulating malignancy: A report on two cases with light microscopy, transmission electron microscopy and immunohistochemical investigation. *Virchows Arch Pathol Anat* 403:391–400, 1984.

67. Zajdela A, Ghossein NA, Pilleron JP, Ennuyer A: The value of aspiration cytology in the diagnosis of breast cancer: Experience at the Fondation Curie. *Cancer* 35:499–506, 1975.

6

Common Breast Carcinomas

INTRODUCTION

About 135,900 newly diagnosed breast carcinomas and 42,300 deaths from this disease occur annually in the United States. In women of all ages, this leading cause of cancer mortality results in 18.8 percent of all cancer deaths. Among 50 countries worldwide, the United States ranks 16th in the age-adjusted death rate from breast cancer; Malta is number one, followed by Great Britain, the Netherlands, and Belgium.[41] It has been estimated that 1 of 11 women will develop breast cancer during their lifetime.[33] Although the incidence has risen over the past 30 years, mortality rates have remained remarkably constant.

Breast carcinoma is found in women of all ages, but is most prevalent between the ages of 40 and 60 and is relatively rare prior to age 30. The risk of developing carcinoma steadily increases up to age 50, then plateaus, and once again rises after the age of 55. In 1,000 consecutive cases of invasive carcinoma, Fisher et al.[17] found that 56 percent were in women 55 years or older and that the incidence was approximately equal in the 20- to 44-year age group and the 45- to 54-year age group. In the younger population, however, they reported that the tumors were probably more aggressive both by biologic behavior and by histologic grade. By contrast, Bloom[6] found an even distribution of low- and high-grade tumors among all age groups.

The risk factors for developing carcinoma are somewhat obscure. Late menarche and early menopause are associated with lower risks, presumably due to a decreased period of ovarian hormonal activity. Obesity and increased dietary fat are considered deleterious factors because they may increase estrogen production. The incidence of breast carcinoma during pregnancy is very low, approximating 3 per 10,000 cases.[46] Nevertheless, the mechanisms of estrogen relationship to the carcinoma are poorly understood. Familial breast cancer tends to occur at an earlier age and is more commonly bilateral than in the general population. In a group of 138 women with breast carcinoma, 38 percent had at least one relative with the disease.[8] Anderson[1] estimated that women with a family history had a 23 percent lifetime probability of developing the cancer, which rose to 27 percent when a first-degree relative was affected.

85

The risk of contralateral breast carcinoma is five to seven times the risk of an initial breast carcinoma and is higher in the younger age group. In Robbins and Berg's[36] 20-year study of 1,458 patients, 6.5 percent developed bilateral carcinoma, an incidence of 7 per 1,000 patients at risk. Leis[28] reported that of 835 patients with unilateral cancer, 9.3 percent had occult contralateral carcinoma diagnosed by random biopsy. Additionally, of 112 patients in good health considered a high-risk group (defined as those under the age of 50 with lobular carcinoma-in-situ, a family history of breast cancer, or nulliparity), carcinoma was discovered in 16.9 percent of those who had undergone prophylactic contralateral mastectomies (see section on "High Risk Lesions" in Chapter 12).

"Multicentricity" refers to the presence of two or more distinct carcinomas within one breast, separated by at least 5.0 cm. Multifocality, by contrast, refers to the presence of several tumors within a single biopsy specimen. Fisher et al.[16] found multicentric tumors in 13.4 percent of 904 mastectomy specimens, one-third being invasive and the remainder in situ. Multicentricity was more frequent with large, stellate tumors, nipple involvement, and intraductal components but had no relation to age, histologic type, grade, nodal status, or lymphatic invasion.

The presence of estrogen receptors and progesterone receptors in malignant cells correlates with the tumor response to endocrine treatment and the prognosis. Up to two-thirds of patients with estrogen receptor–positive tumors respond to therapy with longer disease-free intervals. This interval is significantly increased with tumors positive for both receptors. Estrogen receptor–negative neoplasms are usually poorly differentiated and frequently recur sooner, as well as in visceral sites[7,11] (see Chapter 11).

Clinically, carcinoma of the breast characteristically is palpated as a dominant, stony-hard mass. Gradually, there is fixation with dimpling of the overlying skin. Nipple retraction occurs due to periductal invasion of the tumor toward the nipple. In advanced lesions, the skin becomes thickened and ulcerated.

There are a number of systems for typing malignant tumors. The classification advocated by the World Health Organization,[47] based on morphology rather than histogenesis, is used in this textbook. Many neoplasms are not homogeneous, but rather exhibit combinations of growth patterns, 32 percent in the series of Fisher et al.[17] For nomenclature, the predominant component should compose at least 75 percent of the entire tumor.

The histologic characteristics and degree of anaplasia are major factors in survival and prognosis and are applicable to all types of carcinomas. These include the amount of tubule formation, size and shape of the cells and nuclei, degree of hyperchromatism, and number of mitoses.[6] Nuclear grading, as popularized by Black et al.,[5] has three subcategories, with grade I nuclei indicating the worst prognosis:

Grade I nuclei: Large, pleomorphic macronucleoli; frequent mitoses
Grade II nuclei: Intermediate
Grade III nuclei: Small, uniform, inconspicuous nucleoli; rare mitoses

In the series of Fisher et al.,[17] approximately half had grade II nuclei, about a third were poorly differentiated, and the remainder were well differentiated. Fisher et al.'s 1984 modification[19] of tumor scoring utilizes tubular formation with nuclear grade to form a histologic grade, with grade I tumors giving the best prognosis:

Grade I tumors: Marked tubule formation

Grade II tumors: Complex or moderate tubule formation; or no tubules; uniform nuclei

Grade III tumors: No tubules; pleomorphic nuclei

Utilization of this scheme for 614 carcinomas resulted in an incidence of 11 percent grade I tumors, 23 percent grade II tumors, and 66 percent grade III tumors.

Staging determines the anatomic extent of the primary carcinoma. It is most precise when utilizing the tumor diameter size (T), axillary lymph node involvement (N) and metastatic spread (M)[4]:

Stage I: Tumor <2 cm; no nodal involvement $(T_1N_0M_0)$

Stage II: Tumor 2–5 cm; with or without axillary nodal tumor $(T_2N_0M_0$ or $T_1N_1M_0)$

Stage III: Tumor >5 cm; with or without axillary nodal tumor, without distant metastases $(T_3N_1M_0)$

Stage IV: Tumor of any size; with distant metastases and/or direct extension to the chest wall $(T_4N_1M_1)$

The prognosis is predicted by the presence of tumor cells within the vessels of the breast, as well as in axillary nodes. Tumor-laden lymphatics of the breast are unfavorable. This has been reported in 10 to 15 percent of patients without node metastases.[37,38] In one study of patients with stage I disease and lymphatic invasion, the recurrence rate was 32 percent compared to 10 percent with no lymphatic tumor emboli.[39] Blood vessel invasion has also been related to earlier recurrence and a poorer prognosis. Probably the gravest prognostic indicator is nodal metastasis involving four or more axillary lymph nodes and is associated with relapse and short-term treatment failure.[17] Among 171 such patients, 69 percent suffered treatment failure within 5 years,[18] and after 10 years 71 percent had recurrent disease.[19]

INFILTRATING DUCTAL CARCINOMA

Clinical and Pathologic Findings

This most common carcinoma constitutes about 80 percent of all malignant tumors of the breast.[17] It occurs most frequently in the sixth decade but has been reported from the twenties to the nineties. In the review of Fisher et al.,[17] approximately one-third had heterogeneous components, 50 percent had tubular features, and 6 percent had invasive lobular carcinoma.

About two-thirds of the tumors are stellate, with infiltrating borders. Most of the remainder are circumscribed, with rounded or smooth pushing borders, and a few have indistinct borders. The stellate tumors tend to be larger and are more likely to have axillary lymph node metastases than those with circumscribed margins.[10]

Microscopically, the malignant cells are arranged in cords of two to three layers, nests, large sheets, tubules, acini, or, frequently, mixtures of all types. Well-differentiated carcinoma is composed of uniform cells approximating those of benign ducts. These cells have a relatively normal nuclear/cytoplasmic ratio and round nuclei with inconspicuous nucleoli. In poorly differentiated tumors, the malignant cells are large and pleomorphic, with little or no cytoplasm, hyperchromatic nuclei, macronucleoli, and frequent mitoses. Between the two extremes, the malignant cells are enlarged but relatively regular, with vesicular oval nuclei, some nucleoli, and a few mitotic figures.

The stroma reacts to the infiltrating malignant cells by producing increased amounts of fibroblastic tissue. The stroma may be reduced to a few collagen fibers or may consist of a large, homogeneous mass of collagen tissue which compresses the tumor cells (scirrhous carcinoma). The incidence of scirrhous infiltrating ductal carcinoma is about 3.5 percent.[45]

The histologic and nuclear grades of the ductal carcinoma coincide quite reliably with the prognosis. It has been demonstrated that patients with poorly differentiated ductal carcinoma without tubular features have more and earlier axillary lymph node metastases and, ultimately, more tumor deaths than those with low-grade carcinoma.[20] Patients with an intraductal tumor component reportedly have fewer nodal metastases and a better prognosis.[42]

Lymphoplasmacytic stromal infiltration occurs in about 20 percent of the ductal carcinomas. Lymphocytes are usually more numerous than plasma cells, an infiltrate often indicating an aggressive tumor which is hormone receptor negative. Some investigators, however, have reported that this host response indicates a relatively favorable prognosis.[44]

ABC

Grittiness is encountered upon needle penetration into the ductal carcinoma. Compared to other malignant breast neoplasms, diagnosis of this carcinoma usually is made more easily by ABC because it is based on all the criteria of malignancy. The cell-rich aspirates are composed principally of dyshesive clusters. For those accustomed to interpretation of exfoliated cells, the sea of bland, similar cells with abundant cytoplasm and finely granular chromatin constitutes a seemingly benign appearance. This monomorphism, however, is a prominent malignant criterion of infiltrating ductal carcinoma (see Figs. 6.19 and 6.20).

Dyshesive aggregates of moderate-sized cells characterize the neoplasm. Cell clusters vary from the preponderant small, piled groups to minimally dyshesive, multilayered sheets of up to 50 cells, and a few isolated cells are found. The columnar, oval, or plasmacytoid cells range from 10 to 20 μm in size, with a few as small as 7 μm and a few larger than 25 μm. They display a modest amount of poorly delineated cytoplasm and eccentric, vesicular nuclei ranging from 9 to 12 μm. The nuclear/cytoplasmic ratio approximates 85 to 90 percent,[24] although rarely there is only a cytoplasmic rim. The nuclei show considerable anisonucleosis and irregular, thickened membranes. The chromatin pattern usually is finely granular but may be coarsely granular, with a few atypical mitoses. There are macronucleoli in about 25 percent of the cases (see Table 6.1).

The degree of dyshesion and nuclear alteration depends on the differentiation of the carcinoma. In poorly differentiated tumors there are many small, dyshesive groups and isolated cells. The cells are pleomorphic, with little cytoplasm, marked anisonucleosis and nuclear membrane irregularity, and many macronucleoli. Cellularity and monomorphism remain constant (Figs. 6.1 to 6.5).

There may be microcalcifications. These rounded or irregularly shaped, darkly staining, homogeneous bodies range from 25 to 50 μm. They may be isolated or occur amid a nest of tumor cells (Fig. 6.6). They are pathognomonic for neither ductal carcinoma nor malignant tumors. In nonpalpable lesions, their presence should be indicated (see Chapter 10).

The incidence of falsely negative aspirates from this lesion is low. Most are due to geographic misses because of the tiny size of the carcinomas. In a few cases, the scirrhous component minimizes the release of tumor cells (Fig. 6.7).

In a series of 1,317 ductal carcinomas, Eisenberg et al.[15] diagnosed 69 percent as positive. At our institution over a 3-year period, we classified the tumor type in 86 percent of the 179 palpable and nonpalpable ductal carcinomas interpreted as positive; 9 percent (19) were considered suspicious; and there were 7 percent (16) false-negative cases (Figs. 6.8 and 6.9).[24]

LOBULAR CARCINOMA

Clinical and Pathologic Findings

Lobular carcinoma is the second most frequently encountered carcinoma of the breast. It constitutes about 5 percent of all breast carcinomas as a homogeneous tumor, while in mixed types the incidence rises to 9 percent.[17] Although in one series[17] it was more frequent in premenopausal patients, in our experience and that of others,[30] it is commoner in the older age group. Among 176 patients, the age range was 31 to 96, with a mean age of 52 years, and 22 percent developed contralateral carcinoma.[13]

Arising from terminal ducts and lobules, the tumor is composed of an array of narrow bands of small tumor cells within a dense fibrous matrix. They encircle benign ductal epithelium in a targetoid pattern and extend diffusely into adjacent tissue in Indian file, cords, or singly. Additionally, there are dilated lobules packed with neoplastic cells (in situ lobular carcinoma). The relatively uniform cells with scant cytoplasm may resemble lymphocytes or display a modest amount of cytoplasm, sometimes with globules of mucin. Mitoses are few, and there is little necrosis. Variations of this pattern occur, and in one study only 62 percent showed in situ lobular carcinoma.[13,21]

The virulent signet-ring cell carcinoma was classified by Saphir[40] as an unusual form of mucinous carcinoma. Since it generally lacks large amounts of extracellular mucin, it is now viewed as a variant of several histologic types, particularly lobular carcinoma. In these cases, numerous small cells with crescent-shaped nuclei compressed to the cell periphery by mucin characterize the bulk of the tumors.[43] Foci of mucin-positive signet-ring cells (>20 neoplastic cells per high-power field) also have been noted in ductal and colloid carcinomas (see Figs. 6.11, 6.12).[23]

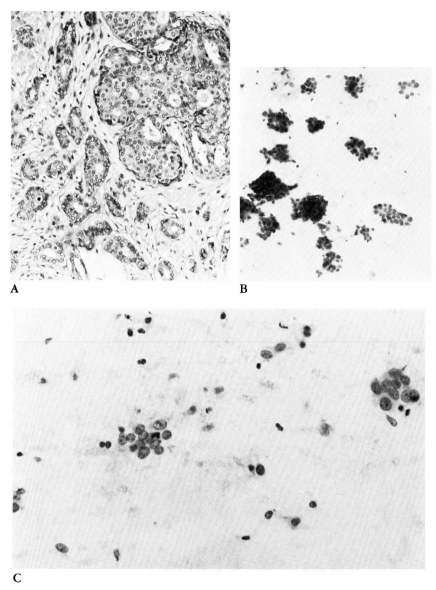

C

Fig. 6.1. Ductal carcinoma, well differentiated. **A.** ABC. Note the uniform cells filling the ducts and infiltrating the stroma. Papanicolaou preparation (×125). **B.** ABC. Note the cell richness with many dyshesive clusters of monomorphic cells. Papanicolaou preparation (×125). **C.** ABC. Note the bland cells with finely granular chromatin. Papanicolaou preparation (×300).

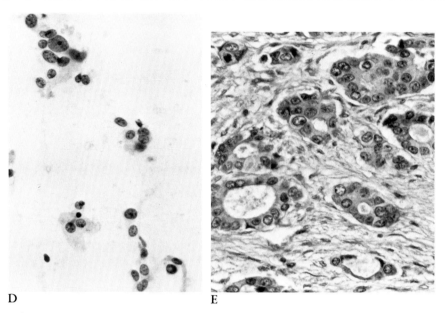

D   E

Fig. 6.1. D. ABC. Note the dyshesive clusters of cells with anisonucleosis and macronu-cleoli. Papanicolaou preparation (×300). **E.** Tissue section. Note the infiltrating ducts with similar cellular features. Hematoxylin and eosin preparation (×300).

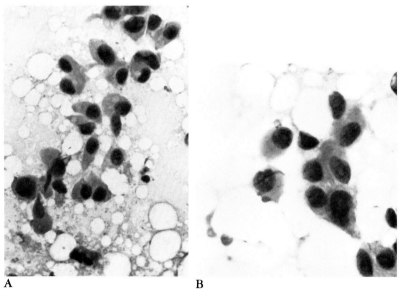

A   B

Fig. 6.2. Ductal carcinoma, ABC. **A,B.** Note the plasmacytoid cells. Papanicolaou prepara-tions (×300, ×500).

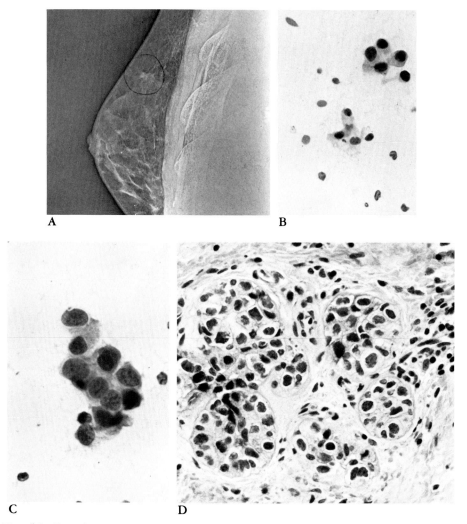

Fig. 6.3. Ductal carcinoma, moderately differentiated; scouting NAB from a 37-year-old woman with a nonpalpable, 0.5-cm tumor. **A.** Mammogram. Note the encircled, superficial irregularity. **B.** ABC. Note the dyshesive, small clusters of cells exhibiting anisonucleosis. Papanicolaou preparation (×300). **C.** ABC. Note the dyshesive group. Papanicolaou preparation (×500). **D.** Tissue section. Hematoxylin and eosin preparation (×300).

Fig. 6.4. Ductal carcinoma, moderately to poorly differentiated. **A.** Tissue section. Hematoxylin and eosin preparation (×125). **B.** ABC. Note the cell-rich specimen composed of dyshesive cords and isolated tumor cells. Papanicolaou preparation (×125). **C.** ABC. Note the dyshesive cord and isolated cells. Papanicolaou preparation (×300). **D.** ABC. Note the marked anisonucleosis, nuclear membrane irregularity, and macronucleoli. Papanicolaou preparation (×500). **E.** ABC. Note the abnormal mitotic figure. Papanicolaou preparation (×500).

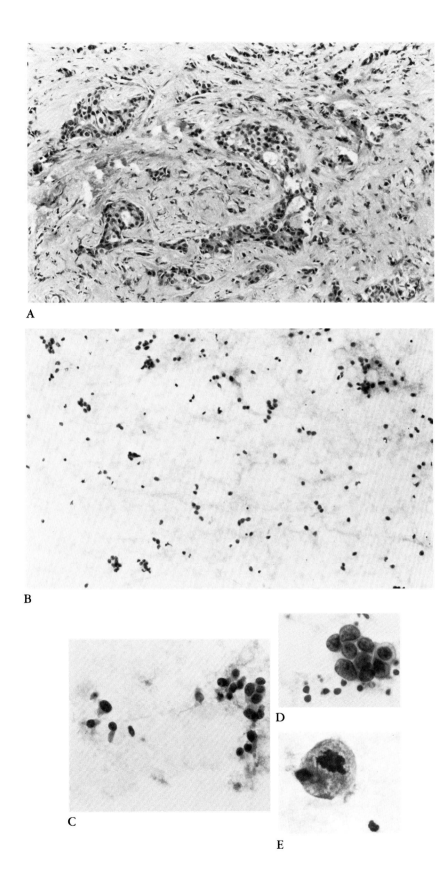

A

B

C

D

E

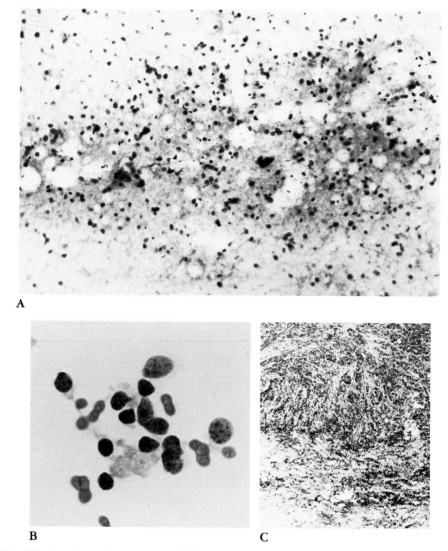

A

B   C

Fig. 6.5. Ductal carcinoma with undifferentiated areas. **A.** ABC. Note the cell density with innumerable isolated cells. Papanicolaou preparation (×125). **B.** ABC. Note the malignant cells, twice as large as adjacent red blood cells, without cytoplasm and with marked nuclear irregularity. Papanicolaou preparation (×500). **C.** Tissue section. Hematoxylin and eosin preparation (×125).

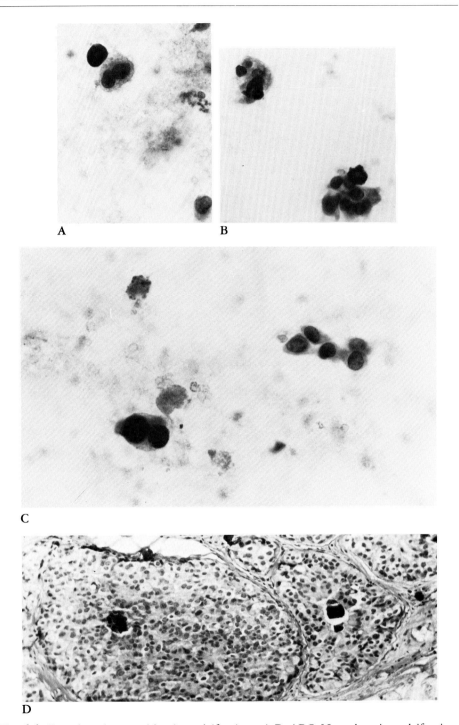

Fig. 6.6. Ductal carcinoma with microcalcifications. **A,B.** ABC. Note the microcalcifications within the cell groups. Papanicolaou preparations (×300). **C.** ABC. Note the microcalcifications isolated as tiny spicules (upper left) and within the cell (lower left). Papanicolaou preparation (×500). **D.** Tissue section. Note the dark calcific bodies. Hematoxylin and eosin preparation (×125).

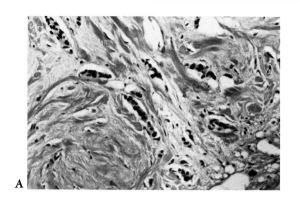

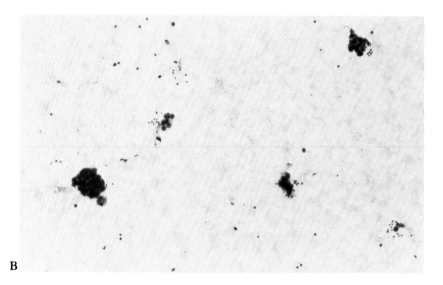

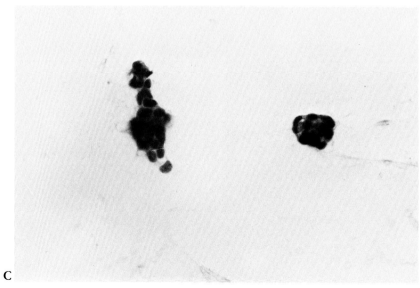

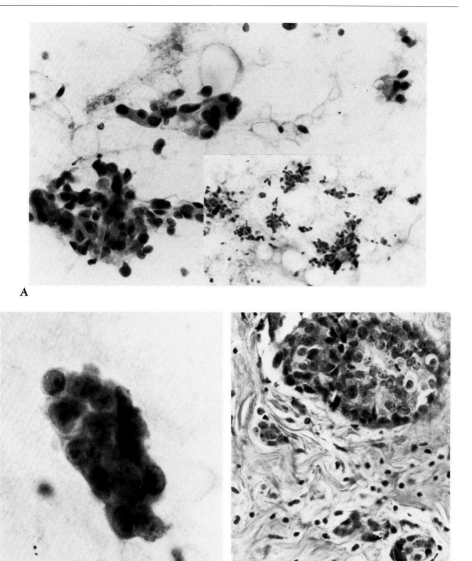

Fig. 6.8. Ductal carcinoma; NAB from a 33-year-old woman during lactation; ABC interpreted as positive. Note all ABC criteria of malignancy. **A.** ABC. Note the dyshesive groups of cells with anisonucleosis. Papanicolaou preparation (×300). *Insert.* Note the cell richness with dyshesive, monomorphic cell groups. Papanicolaou preparation (×125). **B.** ABC. Note the cells with nuclear membrane irregularity and macronucleoli. Papanicolaou preparation (×500). **C.** Tissue section. Hematoxylin and eosin preparation (×300).

Fig. 6.7. Scirrhous ductal carcinoma. **A.** Tissue section. Note the desmoplasia. Hematoxylin and eosin preparation (×300). **B.** ABC. Note the modest cellularity. Papanicolaou preparation (×125). **C.** ABC. Note the relative cohesion of the small groups; these can be mistaken for cells from fibrocystic change. Papanicolaou preparation (×300).

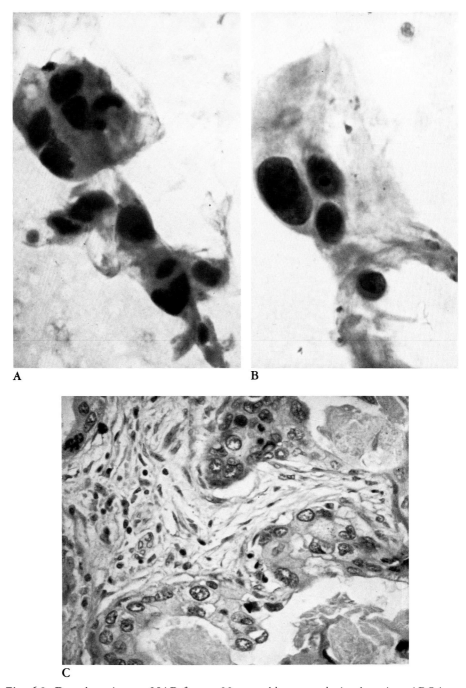

Fig. 6.9. Ductal carcinoma; NAB from a 32-year-old woman during lactation; ABC interpreted as positive. **A,B.** Note the bizarre cells with marked nuclear membrane irregularity, anisonucleosis, and macronucleoli. Papanicolaou preparations (×1250). **C.** Tissue section. Hematoxylin and eosin preparation (×300).

ABC

Lobular carcinoma is the most difficult cancer to detect by ABC because of its often subtle malignant features. The typical pattern is that of a monomorphic, modestly cellular aspirate with small, isolated cells and a few dyshesive groups of no more than 10 cells, either molded or in Indian file. Many times the specimen is cell poor. Four of six randomly selected cases from our files showed fewer than six cell groups on each slide (see Figs. 6.19, 6.20).

The cells commonly approximate lymphocytes in size and appearance. These measure 8 to 12 μm and have only a rim of cytoplasm. They may, however, resemble plasma cells with eccentric nuclei and ill-defined, ample cytoplasm. The hyperchromatic nuclei exhibit inconspicuous anisonucleosis with somewhat uneven membranes. There are macronucleoli in about 25 percent of the cases[24] (Fig. 6.10); (see Table 6.1). Abnormal mitoses are almost never seen. At times, there may be isolated, rounded, basophilic microcalcifications. Koss et al.[26] were one of the first to describe the large intracytoplasmic vacuoles. These may flatten the nuclei to form signet-ring cells or leave them unimpaired. Antoniades and Spector[2] stressed the diversity of the tumor cells, noting nuclei that were round and hyperchromatic, oval or molded with finely granular chromatin, or compressed by sharply defined or bubbly cytoplasmic vacuoles (Figs. 6.11, 6.12).

This lesion causes the majority of false-negative diagnoses. In one review, only 25 percent of 87 cases were interpreted as positive.[15] In one of our studies we interpreted 16 of 35 lobular carcinomas as positive, correctly identifying the dominant tumor type in 75 percent but misclassifying 25 percent as infiltrating ductal carcinoma because of a few dyshesive clusters and some tumor cells measuring up to 20 μm; 12 more were interpreted as suspicious, indicating the need for immediate excisional biopsy; the false-negative rate was 20 percent (7 cases), with no identifiable tumor cells on review.[24]

There are two factors involved in false-negative diagnoses. One is the sparse cellularity due to the dense stroma encircling and confining the malignant cells. The other is the similarity of the small tumor cells to lymphocytes. To detect as many of these carcinomas as possible, we now rapidly review all the slides with the scanning lens after the customary screening. This procedure, which is particularly useful for evaluation of scant aspirates from postmenopausal women, may disclose a few lymphoid cells with abnormal nuclear detail or vacuolated cytoplasm. In the future, the monoclonal antibody B72.3 undoubtedly will shift some suspicious cases into the positive category[29] (see Plate 2.2; the section on "The Surgeon and NAB" in Chapter 8; and Chapter 11).

MEDULLARY CARCINOMA

Clinical and Pathologic Findings

The medullary or soft carcinoma was described in 1949 by Moore and Foote,[31] who distinguished 52 of these tumors in a series of 1,000 carcinomas. Its incidence varies from 4.5 to 6 percent, and about 60 percent are discovered in women prior to menopause. It is more common among blacks than whites.[32] The neoplasms vary

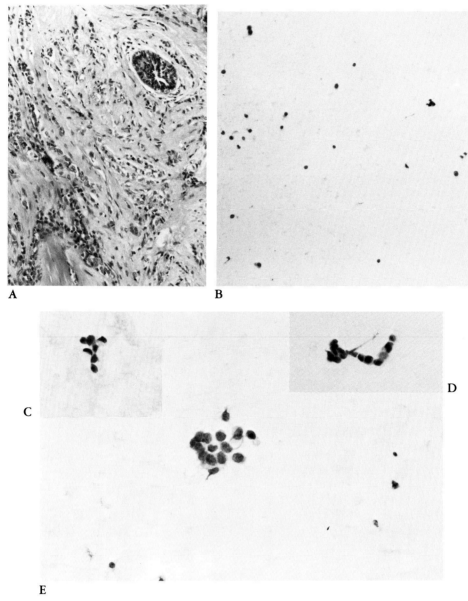

Fig. 6.10. Lobular carcinoma. **A.** Tissue section. Note the small neoplastic cells within a dense fibrous matrix. Hematoxylin and eosin preparation (× 125). **B.** ABC. Note the modestly cellular aspirate with small, isolated cells. Papanicolaou preparation (× 125). **C,D.** ABC. Note the pattern of molded cells and those in Indian file. Papanicolaou preparations (× 300). **E.** ABC. Note the dyshesive group of small cells. Papanicolaou preparation (× 300).

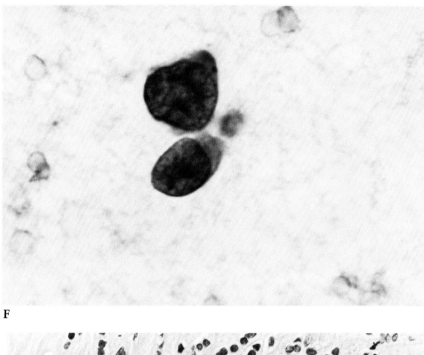

F

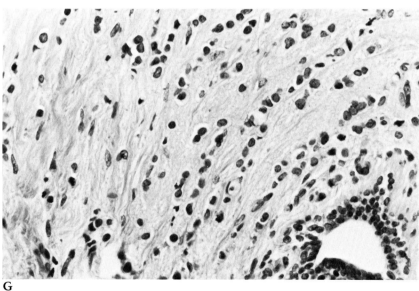

G

Fig. 6.10. F. ABC. Note the cells with a rim of cytoplasmic and nuclear membrane irregularity. Papanicolaou preparation (×1250). **G.** Tissue section. Note the targetoid bands of cells encircling a benign duct. Hematoxylin and eosin preparation (×300).

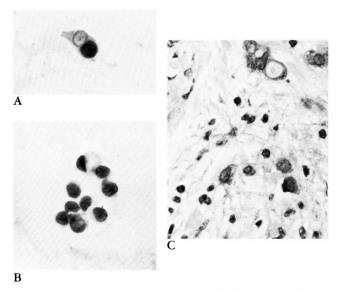

Fig. 6.11. Signet ring carcinoma, lobular type. **A,B.** ABC. Note the small cells with cytoplasmic vacuoles. Papanicolaou preparations (×500). **C.** Tissue section. Note the nucleus compressed by a vacuole. Hematoxylin and eosin preparation (×300).

from 1.0 to 5.0 cm, but large size does not necessarily correlate with metastases. In fact, the 10-year survival approximates 84 percent.[31,35]

The mobile, well-demarcated tumor may resemble a fibroadenoma clinically and mammographically. Grossly, the sometimes bulky neoplasm is characterized by its circumscription. Microscopically, within a dense, mononuclear stromal infiltrate of lymphocytes and plasma cells, the cells form three patterns: the predominating syncytia or solid sheets; trabeculae, consisting of narrow cords less than four cells wide; and aggregates of broad sheets with gland formation. The tumor cells are large, with big, sometimes bizarre nuclei and macronucleoli. Abnormal mitoses are frequent, and in 10 percent of the cases there may be multinucleated giant cells. Calcification is generally absent. Necrosis may be prominent,[17,35] and there may be areas of cystic necrosis.[22] According to Azzopardi,[3] diagnosis is based on the presence of a circumscribed tumor having a syncytial pattern over at least 75 percent of its mass, large malignant cells with pleomorphic nuclei, and a diffuse lymphocytoid infiltrate.

ABC

The aspirate generally consists of a few gray-pink droplets. Occasionally, however, straw-colored or sanguineous fluid is removed. We have examined five such cystic medullary carcinomas.[22]

The ABC is easily interpreted in many instances, both as malignant and as medullary carcinoma. Specific diagnosis is made by the concurrence of three types of cells presenting in various proportions: large pleomorphic cells, bizarre naked nuclei, and

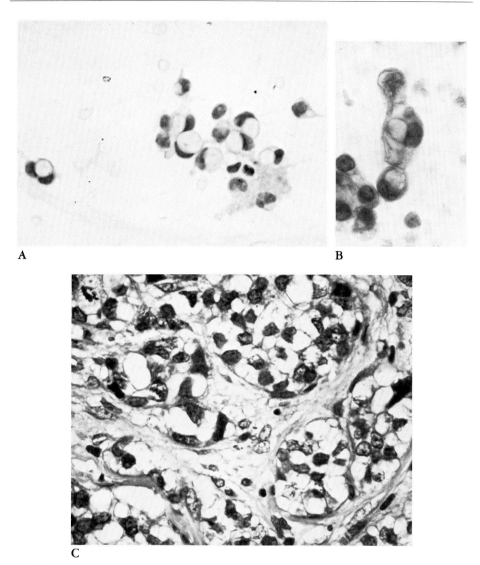

Fig. 6.12. Signet ring carcinoma, ductal type. **A,B.** ABC. Note the dyshesive groups of large cells with signet ring features. Papanicolaou preparations (×500). **C.** Tissue section. Hematoxylin and eosin preparation (×300).

lymphocytes. The cell-rich pattern reveals tumor cells, isolated or in syncytia. Lymphocytes and naked malignant nuclei intermingle to form the diathesis (see Figs. 6.19, 6.20).

The large, pleomorphic cells suggest malignant squamous cells. Often measuring at least 20 μm in their greatest diameter, they form monolayered, nonpolarized, dyshesive sheets (syncytia) of up to 20 cells. The abundant, homogeneous, amphoteric cytoplasm is ill-defined, and the central or eccentric nuclei occupy 60 to 80 percent of the cell volume. The nuclei range from 12 to 15 μm and display membrane irregularity, clumped chromatin, and macronucleoli. Originating from these cells are the identically configured, bizarre naked nuclei. Lymphocytes are scattered throughout in varying numbers[24] (Fig. 6-13; see Table 6.1).

Fluid from necrotic medullary tumors may be more difficult to interpret. The diathesis consists principally of neutrophils with correspondingly few lymphocytes and naked nuclei. Dissociated, bizarre tumor cells are more common than syncytia, and they may be smaller than those from solid lesions. Whenever possible, cell blocks should be made to concentrate the diluted tumor cells[22] (Figs. 6.14, 6.15).

The cytologic literature devotes scant attention to this relatively common tumor. In a 1975 study of seven cases, Zajdela et al.[48] described the cellular pleomorphism and rich lymphocytic population. Eisenberg et al. diagnosed 84 percent of 45 cases as carcinoma, the highest percentage of positive results in their diverse group of neoplasms. Over a 3-year interval, we specifically identified 93 percent of our medullary carcinomas[24] (see Table 6.1).

The preeminence of only one cell form may cause interpretative problems. A preponderance of pleomorphic cells may suggest poorly differentiated ductal carcinoma. Aspirates from the ductal carcinomas (often from postmenopausal patients) display multilayered, dyshesive aggregates instead of monolayered syncytia of the medullary carcinoma. The cells of ductal carcinoma generally are smaller and have less cytoplasm than those of medullary carcinoma, and there are no naked nuclei. From the unusual cystic medullary carcinoma, inflammatory cells may obscure the tumor cells and cause an erroneous diagnosis of benign cyst, particularly in the premenopausal woman. Knowledge of this condition should result in careful examination of all neutrophil-ladened specimens. Furthermore, utilization of the team approach for appreciation of cysts which are incompletely collapsed or recurrent is an important precaution.[22]

MUCINOUS CARCINOMA

Clinical and Pathologic Findings

This carcinoma, also known as "colloid," "mucoid," or "gelatinous carcinoma," was described in 1852 by Lebert,[27] who remarked on its slow growth. It is found in the older age population; the mean age was 63 years in one study.[12] In pure form, it has a frequency of 1 to 2.4 percent, while in combination with other types, notably infiltrating ductal carcinoma, the incidence reaches 6 percent[17,34] (see the section on "Argyrophilic Carcinoma" in Chapter 7). In a 10-year study of 175 patients, survival of those with homogeneous tumors was 90 percent, compared to 66 percent with the mixed type.[25] Controversially, Clayton[12] recommended standard cancer therapy because of his equivocal long-term statistics: 32 percent of 53 patients had cancer-related deaths, many after 11 years, despite a homogeneous tumor and lack of initial axillary metastases. This poor survival may be related to large tumor size, cellularity, and lesser amounts of mucin.[12,25]

Grossly, these often bulky neoplasms are well circumscribed. They are semifluctuant and at least partially composed of a pale, gelatinous substance. Histologically, the masses of mucin, subdivided by loose stromal bands, contain relatively cohesive nests of uniform tumor cells arranged in cribriform pattern, cords, tubules, or papillae. The bland, moderate-sized cells have pale cytoplasm and vesicular nuclei with rare mitoses. Generally, there is neither necrosis nor lymphatic invasion.

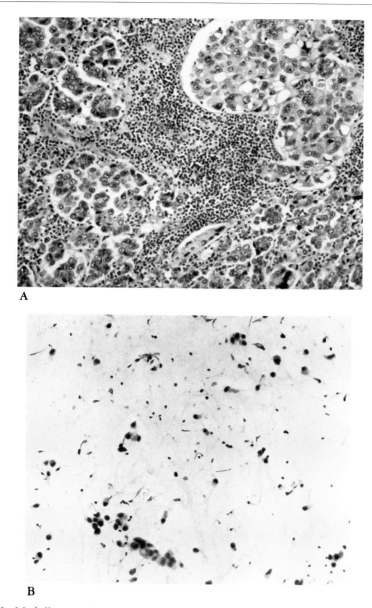

Fig. 6.13. Medullary carcinoma. **A.** Tissue section. Note the tumor composed of syncytia within a dense mononuclear stroma. Hematoxylin and eosin preparation (×125). **B.** ABC. Note the cell-rich pattern of these tumor cells in syncytia and isolated with naked nuclei and lymphocytes. Papanicolaou preparation (×125).

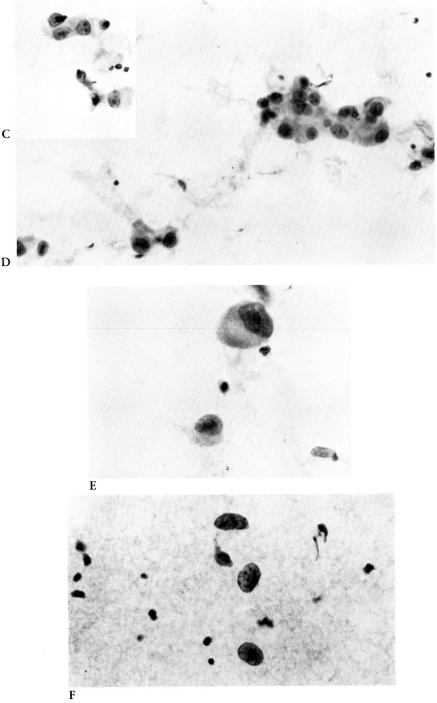

Fig. 6.13. C,D. ABC. Note the dyshesive syncytia of large tumor cells with a sprinkling of lymphocytes. Papanicolaou preparations (×300). **E. ABC.** Note the tumor cells with abundant homogeneous cytoplasm and nuclei exhibiting irregular membranes and macronucleoli. Papanicolaou preparation (×500). **F. ABC.** Note the bizarre naked nuclei with scattered lymphocytes. Papanicolaou preparation (×500).

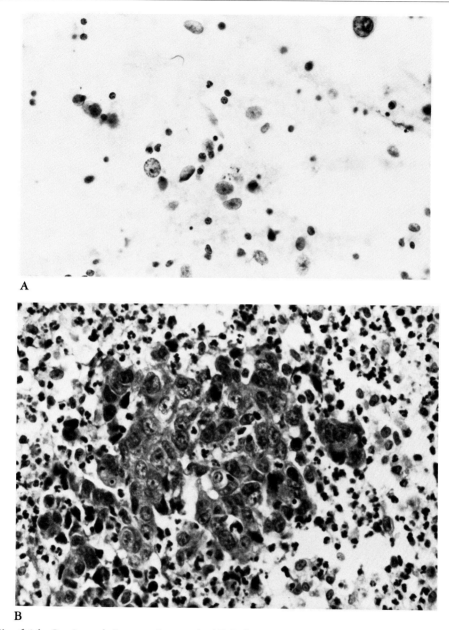

Fig. 6.14. Cystic medullary carcinoma. **A.** ABC, direct smear. Note the chiefly naked nuclei with a bizarre cell (upper right) amid lymphocytes. Papanicolaou preparation (×300). **B.** ABC, cell block. Note the concentration of tumor cells surrounded by debris. Hematoxylin and eosin preparation (×500).

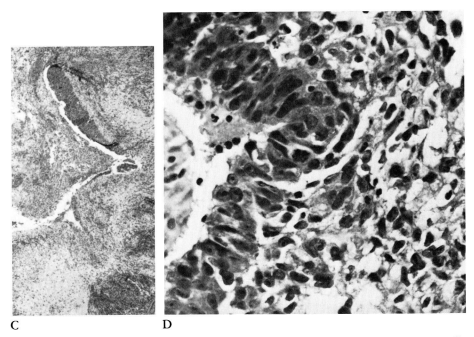

C   D

Fig. 6.14. C. Tissue section. Note the cyst lined by tumor cells (upper right). Hematoxylin and eosin preparation (×125). **D.** Tissue section. Note the tumor cells adjacent to the cyst (left). Hematoxylin and eosin preparation (×500).

ABC

The appearance of the specimen can be diagnostic. It may be glistening, mucoid, and stringy, or it may plug the fine needle. At other times, however, even upon perusal of the ABC, specific interpretation of the carcinoma is elusive.

The cell-rich aspirate displays any of three patterns. The most specific one consists of balls or monolayered sheets of 50 to 500 relatively cohesive tumor cells embedded in thick mucin; additionally, there are scattered, dissociated groups and isolated cells. In the second pattern, dyshesive, monolayered sheets of monomorphic cells in a faintly mucoid diathesis make exact diagnosis more difficult. The third and least specific pattern resembles that of infiltrating ductal carcinoma, which often is a component of this neoplasm. These aspirates, chiefly consisting of moderate-sized cells in dyshesive groups, on careful analysis reveal a few aggregates resting on small strands of mucin.

The common denominator of all three patterns is the mucin. Whether it binds the cells together or constitutes the diathesis, it is the essential ingredient for specific diagnosis. The diffuse or strand-like mucin assumes a pale pink or gray-blue hue with the Papanicolaou stain. In cases with a hemorrhagic diathesis, the mucin appears homogeneous and yellow-orange, resembling colloid. With the May-Grünwald-Giemsa stain it is a vivid pink or violet.[48] In doubtful cases, reactivity to the mucicarmine stain can be confirmatory (see Plates 1.1 and 1.2 and the section on "Stains" in Chapter 2).

The monomorphic cells from mucinous carcinoma are relatively uniform and

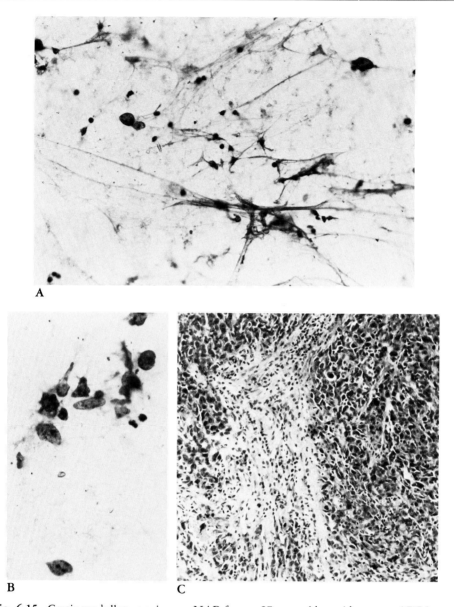

Fig. 6.15. Cystic medullary carcinoma; NAB from a 27-year-old gravid woman; ABC interpreted as suspicious. **A.** ABC. Note the modest cellularity with a few pleomorphic naked nuclei and lymphocytes. Papanicolaou preparation ($\times 300$). **B.** ABC. Note the bizarre naked nuclei. Papanicolaou preparation ($\times 500$). **C.** Tissue section. Note the syncytia and stroma of mononuclear cells. Hematoxylin and eosin preparation ($\times 125$). (Case courtesy of W. David Couch, M.D., St. Joseph's Hospital, Tucson, Arizona.)

bland. They approximate the size of cells from infiltrating ductal carcinoma, measuring from 10 to 20 μm. The cytoplasm is wispy, with ill-defined margins, while the vesicular nuclei, measuring from 6 to 12 μm, display mild anisonucleosis and almost no macronucleoli. Naked nuclei are unusual (Figs. 6.16 to 6.18).

The inconspicuous nuclear alterations plus the cohesive cell balls may suggest a benign process. In these cases, however, the mucinous background, abundant cellularity, disarray of the sheets, and isolated cells should prevent a false-negative report. Cardozo[9] delightfully described the pathognomonic balls as "dark blue islets floating in the large pink colloid mass." In a study contrasting the ABC of mucinous carcinoma with those of other lesions of the breast, Duane et al.[14] reported that the nuclear size (nuclear axis product) was significantly larger than in the benign lesions. In a series of 12 cases, Eisenberg et al.[15] identified 7 as malignant. We interpreted 9 of 10 mucinous carcinomas as carcinoma and one as suspicious; initially, however, only 3 were designated correctly, while the remainder were classed as ductal carcinoma. In review, mucin was clearly apparent in 70 percent of the cases and cell balls in 60 percent; additionally, 70 percent showed many isolated cells and some nuclear membrane irregularity, while a few macronucleoli were noted in three cases and rare naked nuclei in four cases.[24] Zajdela[48] reported similar findings in a study of 36 cases (Figs. 6.19 and 6.20; Table 6.1).

TABLE 6.1. Common Carcinomas: Comparative Cytomorphology[24]

ABC	Ductal (30 Cases)	Lobular (15 Cases)	Medullary (10 Cases)	Mucinous (10 Cases)
Pattern				
Cellularity	+4	+2	+4	+4
Dyshesion	+3	+4	+4	+2
Monomorphism	+4	+4	+2	+4
Nuclear alterations				
Anisonucleosis	+4	+2	+4	+2
Irregular nuclei	+3	+1	+4	+1
Macronucleoli	23%	27%	80%	30%
N/C ratio >90%	50%	93%	—	60%
Cytometry				
Cytopl. diam. (μm)				
<10	13%	73%	—	20%
10–15	64%	27%	—	60%
>15	23%	—	100%	20%
Nucl. diam. (μm)				
<9	27%	85%	—	80%
9–12.5	53%	15%	—	10%
>12.5	20%	—	100%	10%
Special features:	Dyshesive aggregates*	Isolated small cells* Cytoplasmic rims	Large pleomorphic cells* Naked nuclei* Lymphocytes*	Mucin Balls (60%)

* 100% of cases.

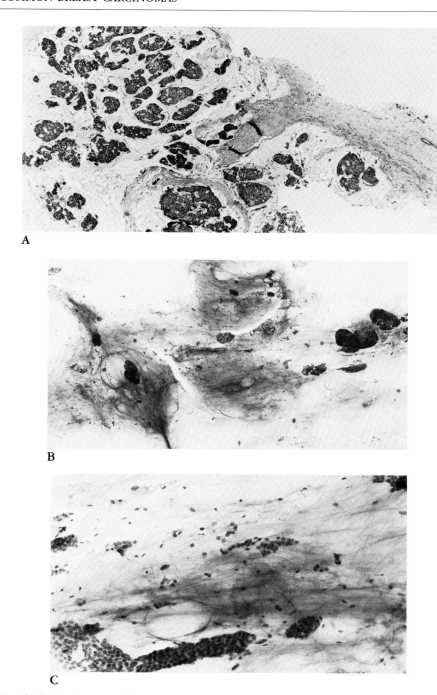

Fig. 6.16. Mucinous carcinoma. **A.** Tissue section. Note the nests of tumor cells within the mucin. Hematoxylin and eosin preparation (×30). **B.** ABC. Note the pathognomonic balls of tumor cells within the mucin. Papanicolaou preparation (×30). **C.** ABC. Note the mucinous diathesis with relatively cohesive sheets and isolated tumor cells. Papanicolaou preparation (×125).

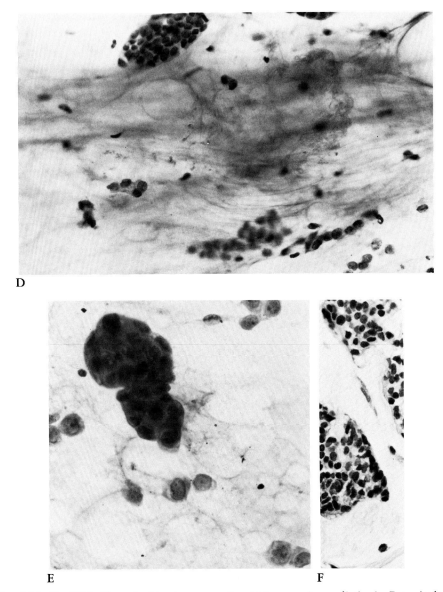

D

E   F

Fig. 6.16. D. ABC. Note the bland tumor cells within a mucinous diathesis. Papanicolaou preparation (×300). **E.** ABC. Note the cohesive ball of tumor cells with adjacent dyshesive, small groups. Papanicolaou preparation (×500). **F.** Tissue section. Note the nests of bland tumor cells. Hematoxylin and eosin preparation (×300).

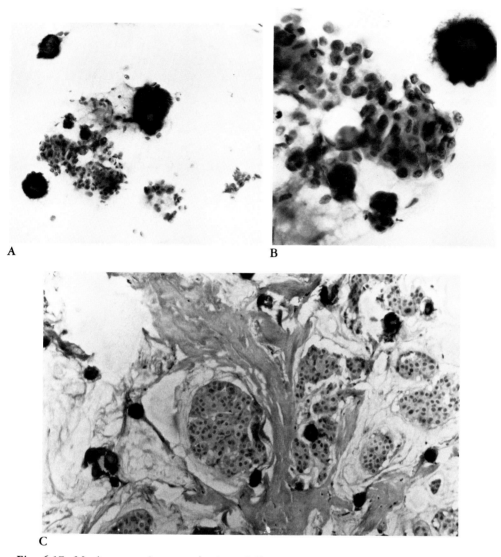

Fig. 6.17. Mucinous carcinoma and microcalcifications. **A.** ABC. Note the microcalcifications embedded in mucin. Papanicolaou preparation (×125). **B.** ABC, higher power. Papanicolaou preparation (×300). **C.** Tissue section. Note the numerous microcalcifications. Hematoxylin and eosin preparation (×125).

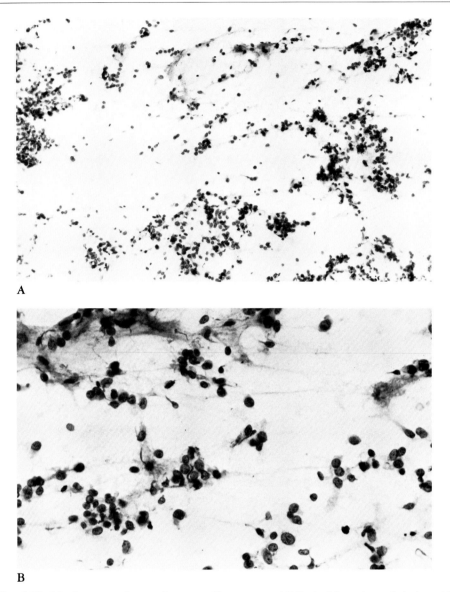

Fig. 6.18. Mucinous carcinoma, least specific pattern, ABC. **A.** Note the cellularity with isolated and dyshesive cells and minimal mucin (upper central area). Papanicolaou preparation (×125). **B.** Note the dyshesive groups and isolated tumor cells with mucinous strands (upper left). Papanicolaou preparation (×300).

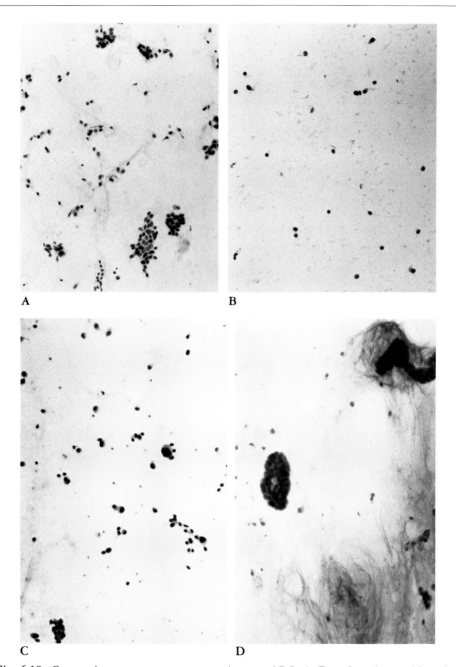

Fig. 6.19. Contrasting patterns, common carcinomas, ABC. **A.** Ductal carcinoma. Note the cellularity with dyshesive, monomorphic groups. Papanicolaou preparation (× 125). **B.** Lobular carcinoma. Note the modest cellularity with isolated cells. Papanicolaou preparation (× 125). **C.** Medullary carcinoma. Note the cellularity with syncytia and a sprinkling of lymphocytes. Papanicolaou preparation (× 125). **D.** Mucinous carcinoma. Note the cell balls with a mucinous background. Papanicolaou preparation (× 125).

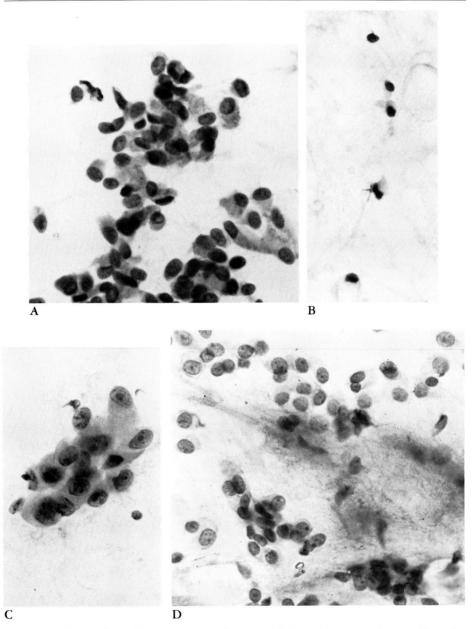

Fig. 6.20. Contrasting cells, common carcinomas, ABC. **A.** Ductal carcinoma. Note the moderate-sized, dyshesive cells with anisonucleosis and rare macronucleoli. Papanicolaou preparation (×500). **B.** Lobular carcinoma. Note the small, isolated cells with irregular nuclei. Papanicolaou preparation (×500). **C.** Medullary carcinoma. Note the large cells with abundant cytoplasm and bizarre nuclei. Papanicolaou preparation (×500). **D.** Mucinous carcinoma. Note the moderate-sized cells with inconspicuous nuclear alterations. Papanicolaou preparation (×500).

REFERENCES

1. Anderson DE: Breast cancer in families. *Cancer* 40:1855–1860, 1977.

2. Antoniades K, Spector HB: Similarities and variations among lobular carcinoma cells. *Diagn Cytopathol* 3:55–59, 1987.

3. Azzopardi JG: *Problems in Breast Pathology.* Philadelphia, WB Saunders Co, 1979.

4. Beahrs OH: Staging of cancer of the breast as a guide to therapy. *Cancer* 53:592–594, 1984.

5. Black MM, Barclay THC, Hankez BF: Prognosis in breast cancer utilizing histologic characteristics of the primary tumor. *Cancer* 36:2048–2055, 1975.

6. Bloom HJG: Further studies on prognosis of breast carcinoma. *Br J Cancer* 4:347–367, 1950.

7. Brdar B, Graf D, Padovan R, et al: Estrogen and progesterone receptors as prognostic factors in breast cancer. *Tumori* 74:45–52, 1988.

8. Bürki N, Gencik A. Torhorst JKH, Weber W, Müller H: Familial and histological analyses of 138 breast cancer patients. *Breast Cancer Res Treat* 10:159–167, 1987.

9. Cardozo PL: *Atlas of Clinical Cytology.* Targa b.v.'s Hertogenbosch, Netherlands, 1973.

10. Carter D. Pipkin RD, Shepard RH, et al: Relationship of necrosis and tumor border to lymph node metastases and 10 year survival in carcinoma of the breast. *Am J Surg Pathol* 2:39–46, 1978.

11. Clark GM, McGuire WL, Hubay CA, Pearson OH, Marshall JS: Progesterone receptor as a prognostic factor in stage II breast cancer. *N Engl J Med* 309:1343–1347, 1983.

12. Clayton F: Pure mucinous carcinomas of breast: Morphologic features and prognostic correlates. *Hum Pathol* 17:34–38, 1986.

13. DiConstanzo DP, Gareen I, Lesser M, Rosen PP: Infiltrating lobular carcinoma (IFLC): A long term follow-up study of 176 patients (abstract). *Lab Invest* 58:25A, 1988.

14. Duane GB, Kanter MH, Branigan T, Chang C: A morphologic and morphometric study of cells from colloid carcinoma of the breast obtained by fine needle aspiration; distinction from other breast lesions. *Acta Cytol* 31:742–750, 1987.

15. Eisenberg AJ, Hajdu SI, Wilhelmus J, Melamed MR, Kinne D: Preoperative aspiration cytology of breast tumors. *Acta Cytol* 30:135–146, 1986.

16. Fisher ER, Gregorio R, Redmond C, et al: Pathologic findings from the National Surgical Adjuvant Breast Project (protocol No. 4); I. Observations concerning the multicentricity of mammary cancer. *Cancer* 35:247–254, 1975.

17. Fisher ER, Gregoria RM, Fisher B: The pathology of invasive breast carcinoma; a syllabus derived from findings of the National Surgical Adjuvant Breast Project (protocol No. 4). *Cancer* 36:1–85, 1975.

18. Fisher ER, Redmond C, Fisher B: Pathologic findings from the National Surgical Adjuvant Breast Project (protocol No. 4); VI. Discriminants for five-year treatment failure. *Cancer* 46:908–918, 1980.

19. Fisher ER, Sass R, Fisher B, and Collaborating NSABP Investigators: Pathologic findings from the National Surgical Adjuvant Project for breast cancers (protocol No. 4); X. Discriminants for tenth year treatment failure. *Cancer* 53:712–723, 1984.

20. Freedman LS, Edwards DN, McConnell EM, Downham DY: Histological grade and other prognostic factors in relation to survival of patients with breast cancer. *Br J Cancer* 40:44–55, 1979.

21. Gad A, Azzopardi JG: Lobular carcinoma of the breast; a special variant of mucin-secreting carcinoma. *J Clin Pathol* 28:711–716, 1975.

22. Howell LP, Kline TS: Medullary carcinoma of the breast: A rare cytologic finding in cyst fluid aspirates. *Cancer* in press.

23. Hull MT, Seo IS, Battersby JS, Csicsko JF: Signet-ring cell carcinoma of the breast; a clinicopathologic study of 24 cases. *Am J Clin Pathol* 73:31–35, 1980.

24. Kline TS, Kannan V, Kline IK: Appraisal and cytomorphologic analysis of common carcinomas of the breast. *Diagn Cytopathol* 1:188–193, 1985.

25. Komaki K, Sakamoto G, Sugano H, Morimoto T, Monden Y: Mucinous carcinoma of the breast in Japan; a prognostic analysis based on morphologic features. *Cancer* 61:989–996, 1988.

26. Koss LG, Woyke S, Olszewski W: *Aspiration Biopsy; Cytologic Interpretation and Histologic Bases.* New York, Igaku-Shoin, 1984.

27. Lebert H: Beitraege zur Kenntnis des Gallertkrebs. *Arch Pathol Anat* 4:192, 1852.

28. Leis HP Jr: Managing the remaining breast. *Cancer* 46:1026–1030, 1980.

29. Lundy J, Kline TS, Lozowski M, Chao S: Immunoperoxidase studies by monoclonal antibody B72.3 applied to breast aspirates: Diagnostic considerations. *Diagn Cytopathol* 4:95–98, 1988.

30. McDivitt RW, Stewart FW, Berg JW: *Tumors of the Breast.* Fascicle 2, *Atlas of Tumor Pathology.* Washington, DC, Armed Forces Institute of Pathology, 1968.

31. Moore OS Jr, Foote FW Jr: The relatively favorable prognosis of medullary carcinoma of the breast. *Cancer* 2:635–642, 1949.

32. Natarajan N, Nemoto T, Mettlin C, Murphy GP: Race-related differences in breast cancer patients; results of the 1982 National Survey of Breast Cancer by the American College of Surgeons. *Cancer* 56:1704–1709, 1985.

33. Ownby HE, Frederick J, Rosso J, et al: Racial differences in breast cancer patients. *J Natl Cancer Inst* 75:55–60, 1985.

34. Rasmussen BB, Rose C, Christensen IB: Prognostic factors in primary mucinous breast carcinoma. *Am J Clin Pathol* 87:155–160, 1987.

35. Ridolfi RL, Rosen PP, Port A, Kinne D, Miké V: Medullary carcinoma of the breast; a clinicopathologic study with 10 year follow-up. *Cancer* 40:1365–1385, 1977.

36. Robbins GF, Berg JW: Bilateral primary breast cancers; a prospective clinicopathological study. *Cancer* 17:1501–1527, 1964.

37. Rosen PP: The pathology of breast carcinoma, in Harris JR, Hellman S, Henderson IC, et al (eds), *Breast Diseases.* Philadelphia, JB Lippincott Co, 1987, pp 147–209.

38. Rosen PP, Saigo PE, Braun DW Jr, Weathers E, DePalo A: Predictors of recurrence in stage I ($T_1N_0M_0$) breast carcinoma. *Ann Surg* 193:15–25, 1981.

39. Roses DF, Bell DA, Flotte TJ, et al: Pathologic predictors of recurrence in stage I ($T_1N_0M_0$) breast cancer. *Am J Clin Pathol* 78:817–820, 1982.

40. Saphir O: Mucinous carcinoma of the breast. *Surg Gynecol Obstet* 72:908–914, 1941.

41. Silverberg E, Lubera JA: Cancer statistics, 1988. *CA* 38:5–22, 1988.

42. Silverberg SG, Chitali AR: Assessment of significance of proportions of intraductal and infiltrating tumor growth in ductal carcinoma of the breast. *Cancer* 32:830–837, 1978.

43. Steinbrecher JS, Silverberg SG: Signet-ring cell carcinoma of the breast; the mucinous variant of infiltrating lobular carcinoma. *Cancer* 37:828–840, 1976.

44. Stenkvist B, Bengtsson E, Dahlqvist B, et al: Predicting breast cancer recurrence. *Cancer* 50:2884–2893, 1982.

45. Van Bogaert LJ, Maldague P: Scirrhous carcinoma of the breast. *Inv Cell Pathol* 3:377–382, 1980.

46. White TT, White WC: Breast cancer and pregnancy. *Ann Surg* 144:384–393, 1956.

47. World Health Organization: The World Health Organization histological typing of breast tumors—second edition. *Am J Clin Pathol* 78:806–816, 1982.

48. Zajdela A, Durand JC, Veith F: Aspect cytologique de quelques variétés particulières d'épithéliomas mammaires. *Bull Cancer* 62:227–240, 1975.

7

Uncommon Neoplasms

INTRODUCTION

The majority of the uncommon carcinomas are constituents of infiltrating ductal carcinoma or have a similar age range and prognosis. Their multiple appellations are indicative of the classification controversy. The neoplasms are described separately, however, because each has a rather distinct ABC pattern. Additionally, a section is devoted to inflammatory carcinomas and cystic carcinomas because of their special clinical presentations, which can be confused with those of benign lesions.

ADENOID CYSTIC CARCINOMA

Pathology

This mammary carcinoma, resembling the salivary gland neoplasm, has an incidence of about 0.1 percent when the histologic criteria are strictly defined. Although it occurs at all ages, it is generally found in postmenopausal women and has been described in men. It most often arises near the nipple. Unlike its salivary gland counterpart, recurrence and lymph node metastases are rarely documented. Therefore, lumpectomy or simple mastectomy may be preferred.[12,83]

Most of these carcinomas are well-demarcated, small, solid neoplasms, but cystic ones have been reported. Microscopically, basaloid cells form trabeculae or cylinders in a hyalinized or mucoid matrix. The cylinders consist of uniform, cuboidal nonsecretory cells in a cribriform pattern or glands of two or more layers with mucoid cores.[12,78] The amorphous luminal material is weakly reactive to mucicarmine and periodic acid-Schiff stains.[54] According to Azzopardi,[5] a biphasic cell population of basaloid and ductal cells is essential for diagnosis. This feature, as well as lack of pleomorphism and luminal necrosis, distinguishes it from intraductal cribriform carcinoma.

121

ABC

The pattern of this tumor is cell rich and monomorphic. There are many small, isolated cells, some acini with mucoid cores, and naked nuclei. Occasional large tissue fragments display sizable rounded, clear, or mucoid pockets.

The majority of the cells are isolated. Measuring from 7 to 15 μm in diameter, some are only minimally larger than lymphocytes. They have ill-defined or barely perceptible cytoplasm and oval, vesicular nuclei 6 to 8 μm in diameter. They show a modest degree of anisonucleosis and hyperchromasia, but inconspicuous membrane irregularity and rare nucleoli.

Some cells are clustered in groups of 10 to 50, with microglandular structures. The latter resemble Call-Exner bodies of the granulosa cell tumor, with luminal mucoid material which is positive to the periodic acid-Schiff and mucicarmine stains (Fig. 7.1). For the few reported cases,[106,108] the Romanovsky technique dramatized the magenta mucoid substance (see Table 7.4).

The differential diagnosis includes infiltrating lobular and colloid carcinoma. The adenoid cystic carcinoma can be distinguished from lobular carcinoma by its cell-dense population and microglandular groups with vesicular nuclei. Distinction from colloid carcinoma is aided by the many single cells, naked nuclei, and absence of cell balls. The rounded, naked nuclei should not be confused with the bipolar ones from fibroadenoma, which also has cohesive fronds; with the pleomorphic ones from medullary carcinoma; or with the elongated ones from papillary carcinoma. Metastatic oat cell carcinoma also must be considered in the differential diagnosis (see Fig. 7.18 and the section on "Secondary Neoplasms" in this chapter).

APOCRINE CARCINOMA

Pathology

The apocrine (sweat gland, oncocytic) carcinoma has an incidence of about 0.4 percent in pure form.[5,38] Although the cells resemble oncocytes, the tumor probably should be classed as a ductal carcinoma. The prognosis is similar, as illustrated in a 16-year matched comparative study of 18 patients.[30]

The carcinoma varies in size from 1.0 to 8.0 cm. It is composed of duct-filled oxyphilic cells which infiltrate the parenchyma. The tumor cells have abundant acidophilic cytoplasm with periodic acid-Schiff–positive granules and vesicular nuclei with macronucleoli. Two essential features are atypical cells and central necrosis.[5]

ABC

By NAB, the lesion is solid. The ABC pattern from well-differentiated carcinoma reveals numerous monomorphic groups of minimally dyshesive apocrine-type tumor cells, chiefly in monolayered large and small sheets. A few form syncytia with little polarity, and there are some isolated cells and naked nuclei. From the poorly differentiated tumor, dyshesion is pronounced, with many isolated cells and naked nuclei. Histiocytes and debris form the diathesis.

The sheets usually consist of 25 to 100 cells, but there may be as many as 1,000.

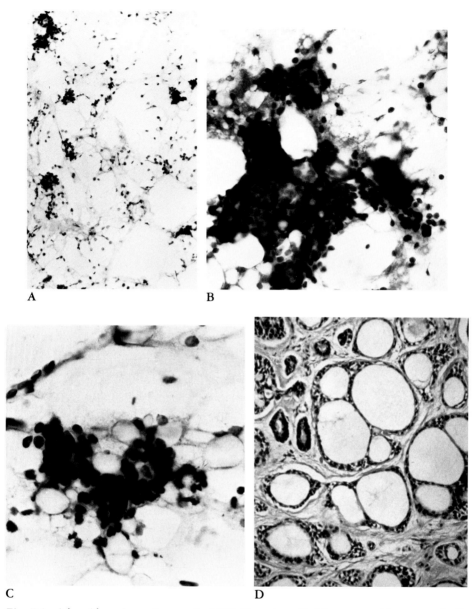

Fig. 7.1. Adenoid cystic carcinoma. **A.** ABC. Note the cell-rich pattern with groups of cells and naked nuclei. Papanicolaou preparation ($\times 125$). **B.** ABC. Note the aggregate with a round lumen corresponding to the mucoid core. Papanicolaou preparation ($\times 300$). **C.** ABC. Note the cells forming microglandular structures. Papanicolaou preparation ($\times 500$). **D.** Tissue section. Hematoxylin and eosin preparation ($\times 125$).

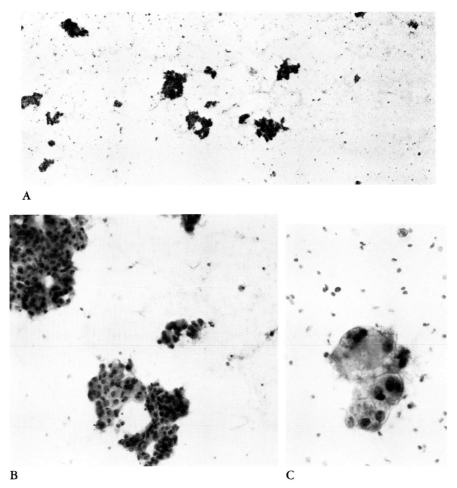

Fig. 7.2. Apocrine carcinoma. **A.** ABC. Note the cell-rich pattern with a diathesis of debris. Papanicolaou preparation (×30). **B.** ABC, higher magnification. Note the monolayered sheets. Papanicolaou preparation (×125). **C.** ABC. Note the group of cells with abundant granular cytoplasm, anisonucleosis, and marconucleoli. Papanicolaou preparation (×300).

The rather uniform cells have indistinct intercellular membranes and vesicular nuclei. They measure up to 30 μm in diameter and have abundant, ill-defined, granular cytoplasm and occasional perinuclear halos. The sometimes multiple nuclei display a modest degree of anisonucleosis, nuclear membrane irregularity, and eosinophilic macronucleoli. The naked nuclei have similar characteristics (Fig. 7.2). A variant with giant, lipid-laden, malignant cells has been described[23] (see Table 7.4).

Aspirates from well-differentiated carcinoma must be distinguished from those of benign apocrine metaplasia. The clinical findings of the former frequently suggest a malignant tumor, and the lesion is solid rather than cystic; the grouped, non-polarized malignant apocrine cells have inapparent cytoplasmic membranes, by contrast to benign cells (Fig. 7.3). Zajdela et al.[106] emphasized the diathesis of necrotic debris.

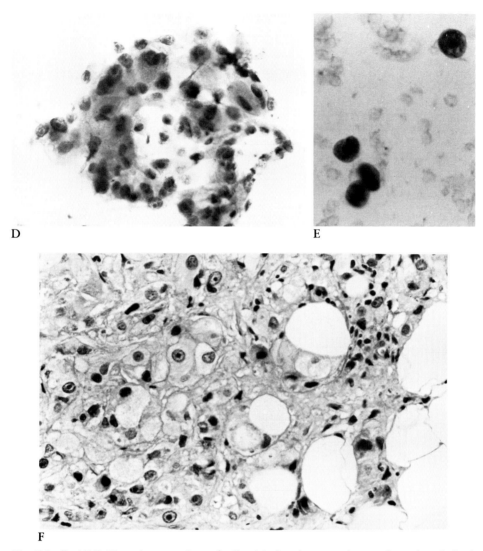

Fig. 7.2. **D.** ABC. Note the syncytium of cells with abundant cytoplasm and poorly polarized vesicular nuclei. Papanicolaou preparation (×500). **E.** ABC. Note the vesicular naked nuclei and debris. Papanicolaou preparation (×500). **F.** Tissue section. Hematoxylin and eosin preparation (×300).

ARGYROPHILIC TUMOR

Pathology

These rare lesions, also known as carcinoids, neuroendocrine or APUD (amine precursor uptake and decarboxylation) tumors, or apudomas, refer to neoplasms arising from diffusely occurring endocrine cells. Some are hormonally active, but all are characterized by certain histologic, histochemical, immunochemical, and electron microscopic findings. These tumors may display argyrophilia (Grimelius

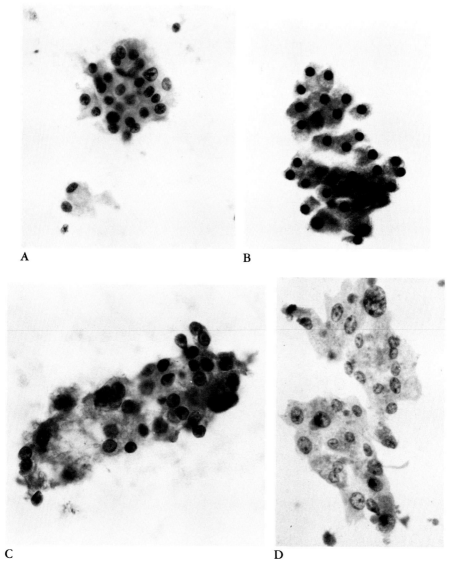

A   B

C   D

Fig. 7.3. Contrasting benign and malignant apocrine cells, ABC. **A.** Apocrine carcinoma. Note the indistinct cytoplasmic membranes. Papanicolaou preparation (×300). **B.** Apocrine metaplasia. Note the distinct cell borders. Papanicolaou preparation (×300). **C.** Apocrine carcinoma. Note the syncytium of cells with macronucleoli. Papanicolaou preparation (×500). **D.** Apocrine metaplasia. Note the marked anisonucleosis and occasional macronucleoli but relatively distinct cytoplasmic membranes. Papanicolaou preparation (×500).

positivity) and/or argentophilia (Fontana-Masson positivity), with cytoplasmic granules which correspond to the ultrastructural dense-core, membrane-bound "secretory granules." These granules probably produce various biogenic amines or regulatory peptides, although many tumors appear clinically inactive.[21]

Microscopically, the neoplasms consist of nests of well-marginated, relatively bland tumor cells within a hyalinized vascular stroma. The small, uniform cells have acidophilic cytoplasm and oval nuclei with small nucleoli. There is scant mitotic activity.

Since several varieties of breast carcinoma may exhibit argyrophilia,[5,77] this tumor classification is controversial. Cubilla and Woodruff,[19] identifying 10 patients with "carcinoid" tumors, reported that their prognosis and metastatic pathway were similar to those of patients with infiltrating ductal carcinoma. While all 10 neoplasms demonstrated argyrophilia and 3 neurosecretory granules, several also showed mucinous features. Fisher et al.[24] found that 8 of 3,300 carcinomas had the morphology of carcinoid tumors, but only 1 exhibited argyrophilia and none argentophilia. By contrast, they identified neurosecretory granules in 19 mucinous carcinomas, 8 of which were argyrophilic positive, and concluded that carcinoid tumor may be a variant of mucinous carcinoma. Taxy et al.[100] similarly observed argyrophilia but no neurosecretory granules in 11 cases. Therefore, the classification of "carcinoid", probably representing a heterogeneous group, should either be eliminated or altered to "argyrophilic tumor".

ABC

The cell-dense ABC is composed of monomorphic, bland cells patterned in monolayered, dyshesive, small and large sheets and isolated cells. The small cells, no larger than 20 μm in diameter, are oval or low columnar in shape. The modest cytoplasm contains granules which may react positively to the Grimelius or Fontana-Masson stains. The vesicular nuclei, occupying up to 80 percent of the cell volume, exhibit minimal anisocytosis and nuclear membrane irregularity. The tumor cells are distinguished from those of ductal carcinoma by their monolayered sheets of uniform cells with vesicular nuclei. (Fig. 7.4; see Table 7.4).

A few cases have been described in the literature, including one from a male breast.[94] The cells with eccentric nuclei have been likened to plasma cells[60] and to lymphoma cells.[73] In a study suggesting the fallacy of the "carcinoid" classification, cytoplasmic argyrophilic granules were observed in both the ABC and histologic sections of two papillary, one mucinous, and two ductal carcinomas.[82]

METAPLASTIC CARCINOMA

Pathology

These rare carcinomas, with an incidence as low as 0.2 percent,[25] comprise neoplasms with features of squamous cell carcinoma, spindle cell carcinoma, pseudosarcomatous tumors, and heterologous tissue (i.e., bone and cartilage). All may originate from focal squamous metaplasia, which is described in about 4 percent of all invasive breast carcinomas,[25] as well as in benign lesions.[72] The majority disclose

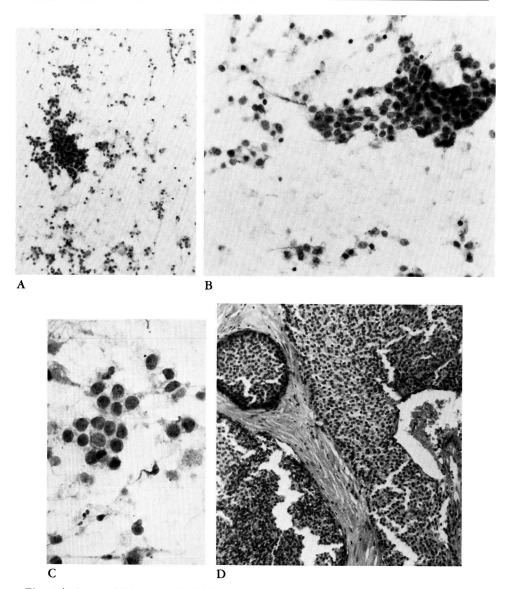

Fig. 7.4. Argyrophilic tumor. **A.** ABC. Note the monolayered, dyshesive sheets and isolated cells. Papanicolaou preparation (×125). **B.** ABC. Note the uniform cells, in sheets and isolated. Papanicolaou preparation (×300). **C.** ABC. Note the bland cells with modest cytoplasm and vesicular nuclei. Papanicolaou preparation (×500). **D.** Tissue section. Note the nests of uniform tumor cells. Hematoxylin and eosin preparation (×125).

remnants of ductal carcinoma upon multiple sectioning. The prognosis is similar to that of other ductal carcinomas and depends on the stage and grade of the tumor.

These large tumors, averaging more than 4.0 cm in diameter, often are cystic, particularly those with components of squamous carcinoma. Most cysts probably are secondary to necrotic tumor, but epidermal inclusion cyst origin also has been postulated.[39]

Histologically, there are various patterns. The most common one is that of infiltrating ductal carcinoma with areas of squamous metaplasia. Some tumors are composed almost entirely of squamous carcinoma with no connection to the overlying skin. Tongues of malignant, sometimes keratinized, squamous cells with intercellular bridges invade a fibroplastic stroma.

Another variety is the spindle cell or pseudosarcomatous carcinoma of epithelial origin, as demonstrated by ultrastructural studies.[72] Bizarre spindle cells display mitotic activity. There may be squamous cell-lined microcysts and heterologous bone, cartilage, or chondroid metaplasia.[72]

Benign multinucleated giant cells, resembling osteoclasts, are found with metaplastic carcinomas and also have been described with ductal carcinoma.[66] Their source has not been established. They may be stromal histiocytic precursors, formed in reaction to the malignant cells,[35,98,102] or they may be related to osteoclasts, even in the absence of heterologous bone.[14]

ABC

The NAB sample consists of droplets from solid portions or turbid fluid from areas of cystic necrosis. Although the ABC reflects the variability of the histology, a specific pattern emerged from a study of 14 cases[53] (Table 7.1).

The ABC is modestly cellular, with a tumor diathesis of necrotic debris, inflammatory cells, histiocytes, and blood. The malignant cells are spindled, squamous, or consistent with those from ductal carcinoma[51] (see Chapter 6). Benign multinucleated giant cells can be seen. Finally, there may be mesenchymal tissue: hyalinized fragments with small, bland, spindled nuclei; cartilaginous sheets; and bony spicules (see Table 7.4).

Benign multinucleated giant cells characterize metaplastic carcinoma. These osteoclastic-type cells, varying from 30 to 60 μm, have abundant, well-delineated cytoplasm and up to 50 central, vesicular nuclei. They are nonreactive to cytokeratin and react positively to S-100 protein and nonspecific esterase.[7,8,35] In some specimens these cells are plentiful, while in others there are few; rarely, they have been described in the squamous cell lesions.[106]

Pleomorphic and bland spindle cells from the pseudosarcomatous metaplastic carcinoma may dominate the ABC. Isolated tadpole or oval cells measuring 15 to 35 μm reveal one or more abnormal nuclei. Smaller, uniform, isolated or bundled spindle cells resemble fibroblasts with regular nuclei and finely granular cytoplasm. Cytokeratin positivity and S-100 protein negativity confirm the epithelial origin of both cell types[7,8,35] (Fig. 7.5; see Plate 1.3).

Squamous cells may constitute the tumor cell population. While many form large, monolayered sheets, others are multilayered and some are isolated. The majority have inconspicuous nuclear changes and resemble mildly dysplastic cells from the cervix. A few, chiefly the dissociated ones, have keratinized cytoplasm with

TABLE 7.1. Metaplastic Carcinoma

Author	Case No.	Fluid	ABC					
			Benign Giant Cells	Malignant Cells				
				Ductal	Bizarre Spindle	Bland Spindle	Squamous	
Boccato et al.[7]	1	0.5 cc turbid	+	−	−	+	−	
Bondeson[8]	2	—	+	+	+	−	−	
Gal et al.[31]	3	20.0 cc turbid	−	−	+	+	−	
Gupta et al.[35]	4	—	+	+	+	−	+	
Hsui et al.[42]	5	—	−	−	−	−	+	
Kline (Current)	6	—	+	−	+	+	+	
	7	2.5 cc cloudy	+	+	−	−	+	
Leiman[61]	8	Small amount, blood-tinged	−	+	+	−	+	
	9	—	−	−	−	−	+	
Oertel[73]	10	Small amount, turbid	−	+	−	−	+	
	11	6.0 cc brown	+	−	+	−	−	
	12	—	+	+	−	−	−	
Sugano et al.[98]	13	—	+	+	+	−	−	
Volpe et al.[102]	14	—	+	+	+	−	−	

Source: Kline and Kline.[53] Reprinted by permission of Alan R. Liss, Inc.

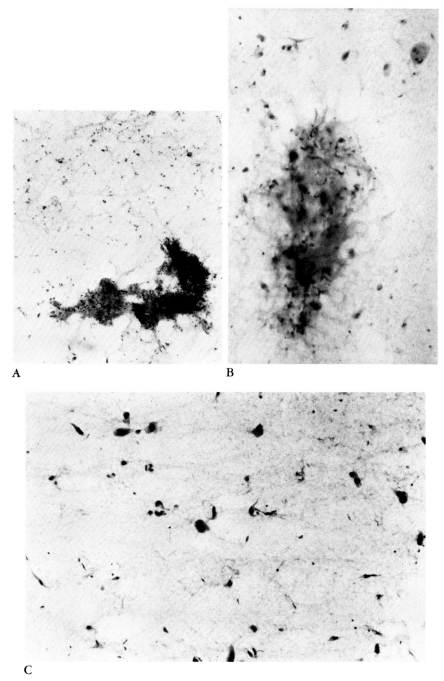

A   B

C

Fig. 7.5. Metaplastic carcinoma, pseudosarcomatous type. **A.** ABC. Note the mesenchymal tissue fragment and tumor diathesis. Papanicolaou preparation (×30). **B.** ABC. Note the mesenchymal tissue fragment and tumor diathesis. Papanicolaou preparation (×125). **C.** ABC. Note the cellularity with isolated spindle cells. Papanicolaou preparation (×125).

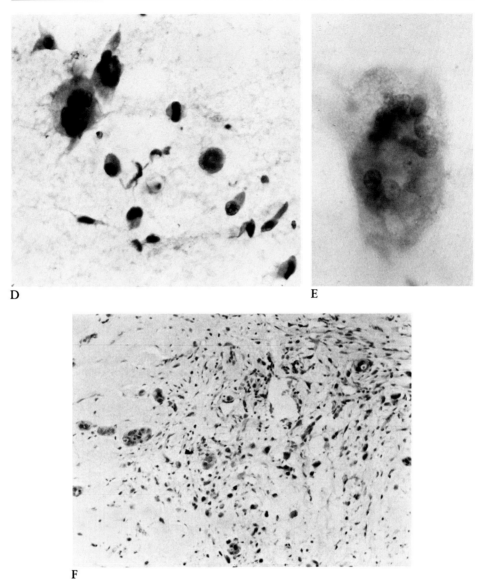

D

E

F

Fig. 7.5. D. ABC. Note the bizarre cells with single and multiple nuclei. Papanicolaou preparation (×300). **E.** ABC. Note the benign multinucleated tumor cell. Papanicolaou preparation (×500). **F.** Tissue section. Hematoxylin and eosin preparation (×125).

enlarged, irregular nuclei, clumped chromatin, and rare macronucleoli. A distinctive feature of the grouped malignant squamous cells is their ill-defined borders.

These tumors may be erroneously interpreted as benign lesions because of cystic specimens containing relatively few tumor cells or because of bland squamous cells. The fluid aspirates may be mistaken for abscess, since tumor cells are masked by neutrophils, necrotic debris, and histiocytes. Furthermore, the dilute, spindled, neoplastic cells resemble fibroblasts, and the osteoclastic-type giant cells suggest an inflamed cyst. Awareness of presentation and pattern will prevent error. In the squamous cell variety, the relatively uniform cells may lead to the faulty impression of a keratinous cyst. The correct diagnosis, however, is indicated by the monomorphism with abundant, indistinctly delineated squamous cells, occasional pleomorphic squamous cells, and tumor diathesis (Fig. 7.6).

PAPILLARY CARCINOMA

Pathology

The homogeneous invasive papillary carcinoma has an incidence of about 2 percent,[26] whereas the intraductal variety has a higher frequency, particularly as a component of other tumors. The average age of onset is 63, although it has been seen from ages 42 to 87.[11] Clinical features include sanguineous or serous nipple discharge[34] and a periareolar mass. The favorable life expectancy of patients with homogeneous tumors equals that of patients with mucoid carcinoma.[26] Eight of 11 patients treated by lumpectomy alone had no recurrence after 10 years.[11]

Papillary carcinomas probably arise de novo rather than from intraductal papillomas. The supposition that the papilloma undergoes malignant change often is based on erroneous diagnosis of the original papillary lesion. McDivitt et al.[65] reported that 12 of 15 patients with papillary carcinoma preceded by "benign papillomas" actually had initial intraductal carcinoma.

Papillary lesions larger than 3.0 cm are usually malignant,[5] and the carcinoma may be as large as 10 cm in its greatest diameter.[56] Grossly, most are circumscribed, cystic masses with foci of hemorrhage and necrosis. Microscopically, there is an arborescent, complex glandular pattern, with solid areas in about one-third of the cases.[11] The multiple stalks have inconspicuous fibrovascular cores and little intervening stroma. Ducts and papillae are lined by monotonous, stratified, columnar or cuboidal cells with little pleomorphism. There may be microcalcifications and necrosis. The monomorphic tumor cells are virtually never interspersed with apocrine-type cells.[5]

ABC

Pink-tinged droplets generally are procured from the carcinoma by NAB. Abundant hemorrhagic or chocolate-colored fluid may be collected from the intracystic form.

The distinctive pattern of papillary carcinoma was delineated in our review of eight homogeneous cases (Table 7.2). The cell-dense ABC consists of papillae,

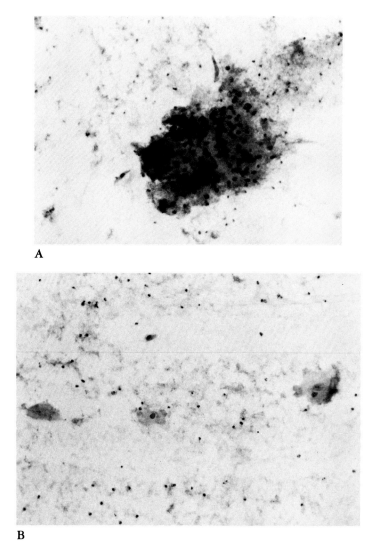

Fig. 7.6. Metaplastic carcinoma, squamous type. **A.** ABC. Note the sheet of squamous cells with ill-defined cytoplasmic borders. Papanicolaou preparation (×125). **B.** ABC. Note the isolated squamous cells in the tumor diathesis. Papanicolaou preparation (×125).

isolated cells including tall columnar ones, and naked nuclei in a diathesis of blood. The cells frequently are bland, with inconspicuous nuclear alterations.

Papillae make up the classic architectural design. These often large, tightly or loosely connected fragments resemble the fronds from fibroadenoma, with finger-like projections and straight or curved margins. Additionally, there are small, dyshesive units of no more than 30 cells.

Tall columnar cells are characteristic of this neoplasm. They may constitute the dissociated cells and also may be distinguished at the periphery of many of the papillae. Measuring up to 20 μm in length, the cells generally are uniform, with moderate to abundant cytoplasm and bland nuclei. The elongated or oval nuclei, ranging from 6

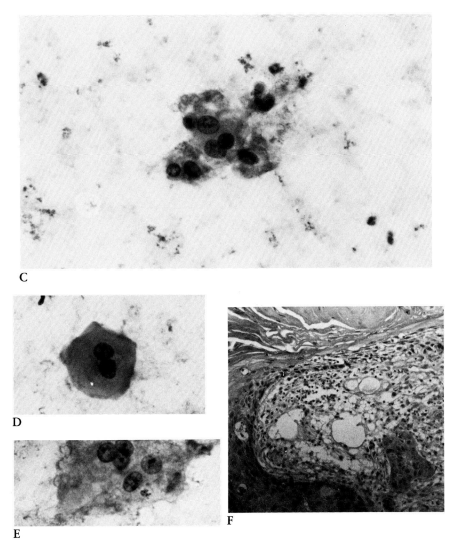

Fig. 7.6. C. ABC. Note the bland malignant squamous cells with indistinct cytoplasmic margins. Papanicolaou preparation (×500). **D.** ABC. Note the multinucleated malignant, keratinized squamous cell. Papanicolaou preparation (×500). **E.** ABC. Note the benign multinucleated giant cell. Papanicolaou preparation (×500). **F.** Tissue section. Note the early cystic necrosis. Hematoxylin and eosin preparation (×125).

to 15 μm in size, display little anisonucleosis, and many have finely granular chromatin. The plentiful naked nuclei exhibit similar features (Figs. 7.7, 7.8).

A sanguineous diathesis is common. Hemosiderin-laden macrophages and necrotic debris may be prominent. Occasionally, blood obscures the underlying cells, and in these cases only a cell block preparation will reveal the diagnostic papillae (Fig. 7.9).

In our cytomorphologic study of papillary carcinoma, there were originally nine

TABLE 7.2. Papillary Carcinoma: Cytomorphology

Cases	Papillae	Isolated Cells	Blood	Tall Columnar Cells	Naked Nuclei
1	+3	+3	+3*	+2	+2
2	+2	+2	+3*	+3	+2
3	+3	+2	—	+2	+3
4	+3	+3	+2*	+3	+1
5	+3	+2	+2	+2	+3
6	+3	+3	+3	+2	+3
7	+3	+2	+3*	+2	+3
8	+3	+3	+1*	+3	+1

*Hemosiderin-laden macrophages.
Source: Kline and Kannan.[50] Reprinted by permission of the American Medical Association.

cases.[50] One of the two cystic tumors, consisting of 15 cc of hemorrhagic fluid, was excluded, however, because only the cell block preparation was adequate; the second, a 0.5-cc specimen, was examined on the direct smear. All eight cases were cell rich, with dyshesive and isolated cells, but in three, nuclear alterations were inconspicuous. Therefore, initially, only half had been interpreted exactly; two, although positive, were incorrectly typed; and two were called suspicious. A similar study confirmed the reproducibility of our findings[69] (see Tables 7.2, 7.4).

Because of the sometimes minimal nuclear changes, the ABC from papillary carcinoma can be misconstrued as a fibroadenoma or papilloma. The fibroadenoma

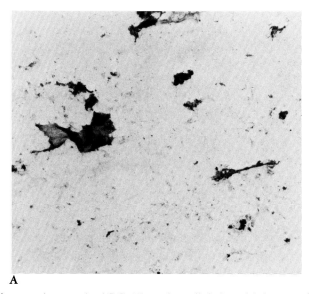

A

Fig. 7.7. Papillary carcinoma. **A.** ABC. Note the cellularity with large and small papillae. Papanicolaou preparation (× 30).

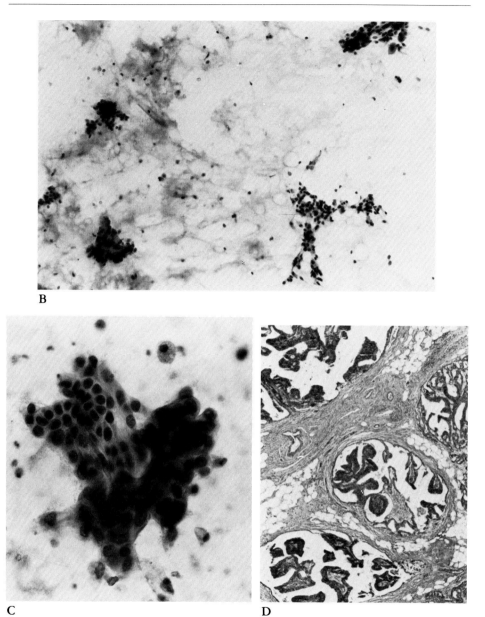

Fig. 7.7. B. ABC. Note the tight and loose papillae and tumor diathesis. Papanicolaou preparation (×125). **C.** ABC. Note the papilla and the tumor diathesis. Papanicolaou preparation (×500). **D.** Tissue section. Hematoxylin and eosin preparation (×125).

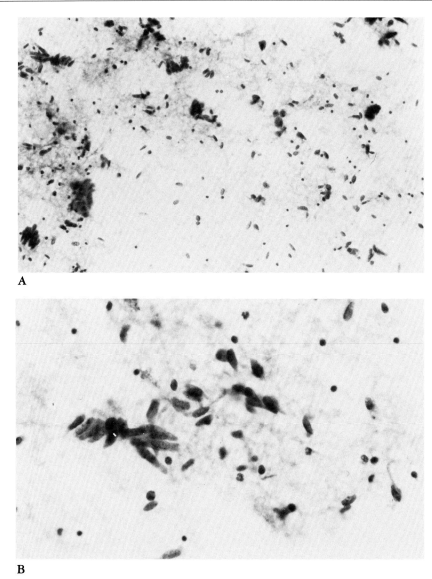

A

B

Fig. 7.8. Papillary carcinoma. **A.** ABC. Note the cell density with small papillae and many isolated cells and naked nuclei. Papanicolaou preparation (×125). **B.** ABC. Note the dyshesive group of tall columnar cells. Papanicolaou preparation (×300).

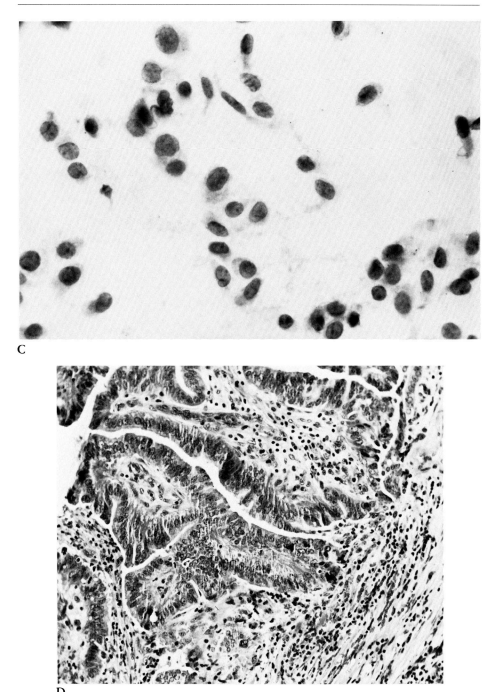

C

D

Fig. 7.8. C. ABC. Note the isolated tall columnar cells. Papanicolaou preparation (×500).
D. Tissue section. Note the malignant papillae of columnar cells. Hematoxylin and eosin
preparation (×300).

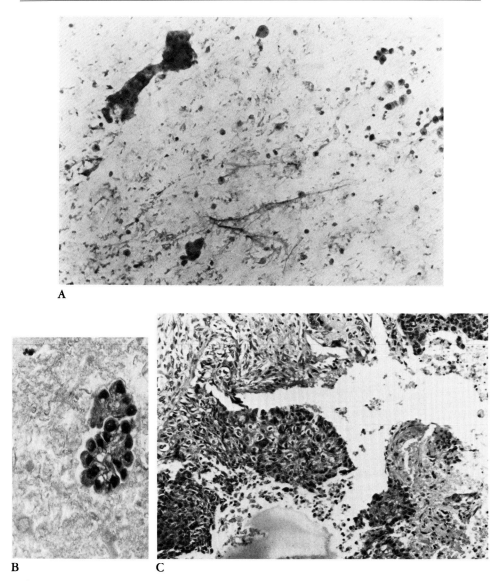

Fig. 7.9. Cystic papillary carcinoma. **A.** ABC. Note the rather degenerated cells in a tumor diathesis, direct smear. Hematoxylin and eosin preparation (×125). **B.** Cell block preparation. Note the papilla. Hematoxylin and eosin preparation (×300). **C.** Tissue section, cystic papillary carcinoma. Hematoxylin and eosin preparation (×125).

is suggested because of the cell richness, frond-like papillae, and naked nuclei. Naked nuclei from the fibroadenoma, however, are bipolar and small (approximately 6 μm), by contrast to the elongated ones (averaging 12 μm) from the carcinoma. Furthermore, small, dyshesive papillae and a hemorrhagic diathesis with hemosiderin-laden macrophages are unusual findings in the benign tumor. The ABC from the papilloma may consist of a few papillae in a hemorrhagic diathesis. Yet, it is relatively cell poor and polymorphic, and in most cases lacks the isolated

TABLE 7.3. Papillary Carcinoma and Benign Lesions: Comparative Cytomorphology

Morphology	Papillary Carcinoma	Subareolar Papillomatosis	Other Papillomas	Fibroadenoma
Cell rich	+	+	−	+
Dyshesion	+	+	−	±
Hemosiderin macrophages	+	±	±	−
Naked nuclei	+	±	±	−
Special features	Tall columnar cells Elongated naked nuclei	Polymorphism Clinical findings	Polymorphism Cell balls	Dimorphism Bipolar naked nuclei

tall columnar cells and bare nuclei. The solitary, large papilloma and florid subareolar papillomatosis may present special diagnostic problems (see the section on "Papillomas" in Chapter 5). In these cases the cell-rich ABC may demonstrate both papillae and isolated columnar cells. Polymorphism, however, is expressed in the form of a few squamous, apocrine, and foam cells, while naked nuclei are unusual; and the clinical presentation of the subareolar lesion is characteristic (Table 7.3 and Figs. 7.10, 7.11; see Fig. 7.18).

SECRETORY CARCINOMA

Pathology

This rare carcinoma goes by a number of names: "clear cell," "lipid-rich," and "histiocytoid carcinoma"; and "signet-ring carcinoma" sometimes is included. The clinical features are nonspecific. Some are reported in the young and others in the aged; the prognosis varies considerably. We shall refer to the entire group as "secretory carcinoma," excluding the signet-ring cell form (see the section on "Lobular Carcinoma" in Chapter 6).

Microscopically, these irregularly marginated tumors consist of solid sheets, nests, or papillae with extra- or intracellular secretions. The polygonal or columnar cells have finely granular, clear, or foamy cytoplasm and vesicular nuclei with rare mitoses. Mucicarmine, periodic acid-Schiff, and oil red O stains, show a variety of responses. Although secretory cells dominate at least half of the tumor, other components, notably infiltrating ductal carcinoma, are often seen.[27,43,99] The differential diagnosis encompasses metastatic adenocarcinoma and renal cell carcinoma.

Fisher et al.,[27] finding 3 percent of 1,550 carcinomas with a clear cell component, concluded that these neoplasms were all variants of well-established carcinoma. They stated that there was a "lack of evidence indicating that the cellular alterations per se have any significant independent influence on survival or that the treatment of these cancers should be different from that of breast cancers lacking these features."

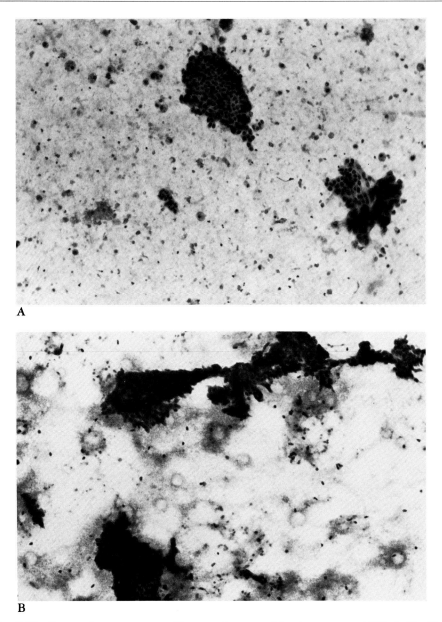

A

B

Fig. 7.10. Contrasting patterns: papillary carcinoma and benign tumors, ABC. **A.** Papillary carcinoma. Note the cell-rich specimen with papillae and tumor diathesis. Papanicolaou preparation (×125). **B.** Fibroadenoma. Note the fronds and naked nuclei. Papanicolaou preparation (×125).

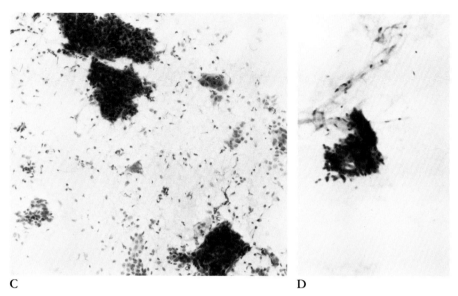

C   D

Fig. 7.10. C. Subareolar papillomatosis. Note the dense cell clusters and isolated cells with few polymorphic groups. Papanicolaou preparation (×125). D. Papilloma. Note the papilla in the cell-poor aspirate. Papanicolaou preparation (×125).

ABC

The pattern resembles that of infiltrating ductal carcinoma. Some cells, however, have distinctively demarcated, clear or vacuolated cytoplasm.

The ABC is cell dense. There are large groups with minimal dyshesion, loose aggregates, isolated cells, and naked nuclei. There may be a few sheets composed of honeycombined, well-delineated, vacuolated cells. Distinctive tissue fragments with cytoplasmic spaces have been described.[3] The relatively uniform cells range from 12 to 20 μm in diameter. Some are oval or polyhedral with pale, granular, or vacuolated, well-defined cytoplasm, while others have scant cytoplasm. The vesicular nuclei exhibit anisonucleosis, minimal membrane irregularity, and a few eosinophilic macronucleoli (Fig. 7.12; see Table 7.4).

The differential diagnosis includes infiltrating ductal, signet-ring, and metastatic carcinoma (see the section on "Secondary Neoplasms" in this chapter). Most reported cases [3,17,70] and one of ours were interpreted as infiltrating ductal carcinoma. In ductal carcinoma, however, the cytoplasm is neither well defined nor vacuolated. In signet-ring carcinoma, the often small cells have ill-defined cytoplasm and crescent-shaped rather than vesicular nuclei (see Figs. 6.11 and 6.12 and the section on "Lobular Carcinoma" in Chapter 6).

TUBULAR CARCINOMA

Pathology

This well-differentiated, invasive, glandular carcinoma generally is found in association with other carcinomas. It is categorized as a mixed tubular carcinoma when the

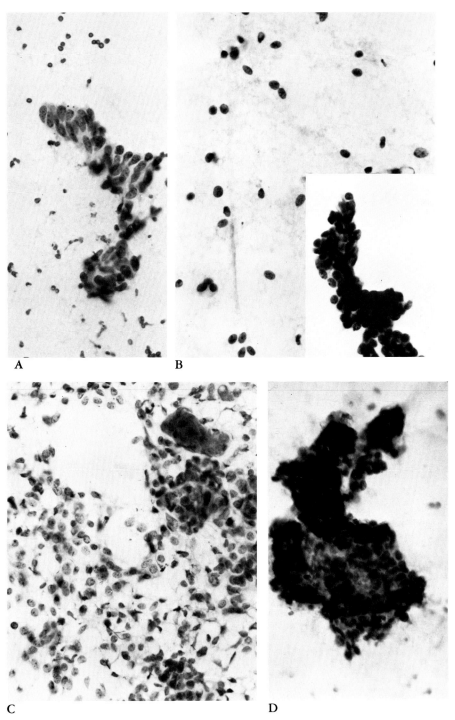

Fig. 7.11. Contrasting cells: papillary carcinoma and benign tumors, ABC. **A.** Papillary carcinoma. Note the dyshesive papilla of tall columnar cells and diathesis of blood. Papanicolaou preparation (×300). **B.** Fibroadenoma. Note the chiefly bipolar naked nuclei and cohesive frond (insert). Papanicolaou preparation (×300). **C.** Subareolar papillomatosis. Note the polymorphism. Papanicolaou preparation (×300). **D.** Papilloma. Note the cohesive papilla. Papanicolaou preparation (×300).

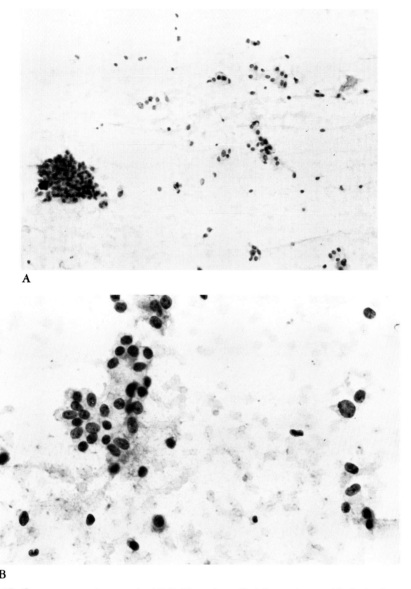

A

B

Fig. 7.12. Secretory carcinoma. **A.** ABC. Note the cell-rich specimen with dyshesive aggregates and isolated cells, a few with well-demarcated cytoplasm (upper center). Papanicolaou preparation (×125). **B.** ABC. Note the sheet of tumor cells with distinctly demarcated cytoplasm. Papanicolaou preparation (×300).

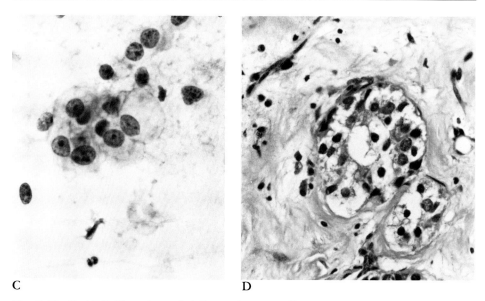

C   D

Fig. 7.12. **C.** ABC. Note the well-delineated tumor cells with clear cytoplasm and vesicular nuclei with macronucleoli. Papanicolaou preparation (×500). **D.** Tissue section. Note the secretory tumor cells. Hematoxylin and eosin preparation (×300).

tubules constitute at least 75 percent of the tumor. In a study of 20 such patients, Carstens et al.[10] emphasized their long-term survival.

Most tumors are small and often adjacent to areas of fibrocystic change. By contrast to sclerosing adenosis, the tumor is infiltrative rather than circumscribed. Widely patent, angulated tubules proliferate in disarray within an abundant fibro-collagenous matrix. The glands are formed by a single layer of bland cuboidal cells without myoepithelial cells.[5]

ABC

Very few of these homogeneous neoplasms have been viewed by ABC. We have seen two cases. Both were characterized by a relatively cell-poor ABC consisting of isolated cells as well as occasional acini. The bland cells, slightly larger than those from infiltrating lobular carcinoma, had scant cytoplasm and vesicular nuclei with finely granular chromatin and minimal anisonucleosis (Fig. 7.13). Others[73,75] have described sheets, tubules, and occasional mucin-filled glands (Table 7.4).

CYSTOSARCOMA PHYLLODES

Pathology

Cystosarcoma phyllodes, a tumor resembling fibroadenoma, has a misleading name, since the vast majority are benign, with some borderline cases and a few frankly malignant varieties. The name "sarcoma" was initially applied because of the tumor's

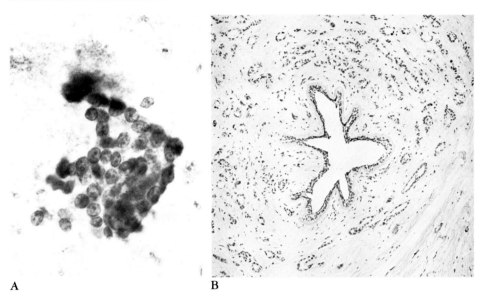

A   B

Fig. 7.13. Tubular carcinoma. **A.** ABC. Note the dyshesive tubular arrangement of small cells. Papanicolaou preparation ($\times 500$). **B.** Tissue section. Hematoxylin and eosin preparation ($\times 125$). (Courtesy of Denise F. Hidvegi, M.D., Northwestern Memorial Hospital, Chicago.)

size and fleshy appearance, with cystic spaces and leaf-like ductal protrusions (phyllodes). At least 90 percent are benign,[5] despite the presence of malignant features in about a quarter.[45] Hajdu et al.[36] reported recurrence in 18 percent of 150 patients with benign-appearing tumors and only 8 percent of 49 with malignant features.

The neoplasm, with an incidence of less than 1 percent, is most frequently found in middle-aged women[5] but occurs from adolescence to old age. Its classic clinical presentation is rapid growth with overlying tense, prominently veined skin.

Grossly, the tumor is spherical, firm, and relatively well-circumscribed, measuring from 1.0 to 30.0 cm in diameter. Although resembling a giant fibroadenoma, its most important differentiating feature is its dense stromal component. This stromal proliferation usually overwhelms the few epithelial structures, but ductal elements must be demonstrated for diagnosis. The stroma is arranged in anastomosing and whorled bundles, sometimes with pronounced intercellular edema. These nodules project into cystic spaces linked by cuboidal or columnar epithelium, giving the appearance of papillae. The stromal cells are large and spindly with pleomorphic nuclei and frequent mitoses. Although the stromal cells are generally fibroblastic in type, lipid cells, cartilage, bone, and squamous metaplasia are found in less than 10 percent of the cases.[71]

Histologic characteristics for predicting biologic behavior include tumor size and contour, necrosis, mitotic activity, and cellular atypia. Pietruszka and Barnes[80] divided their 42 patients into benign, borderline, and malignant subgroups purely on the basis of stromal mitoses. Ward and Evans[103] felt that the stromal overgrowth, with absence of epithelial structures in an area greater than a single low-power microscopic field, was the most significant indicator of a malignant tumor. Clearly malignant tumors have infiltrating peripheral borders and stromal constituents con-

TABLE 7.4. Unusual Carcinomas: Comparative Cytomorphology

Carcinoma	Architecture*				Cells			Nuclei			Special Features
	Fluid NAB	Tissue Fragments	Sheets	Dyshesive Groups	Bland	Size†	Mucin	Naked	Multiple	Macronucleoli	
Adenoid cystic	−	+	−	+	+	S	±	+	−	−	Microglands Mucin
Apocrine	−	−	+	±	−	M	−	+	+	+	Apocrine cells
Argyrophilic	−	−	+	+	+	M	−	−	−	−	Grimelius + cytoplasmic granules
Metaplastic	±	+	+	+	±	L	−	−	+	+	Benign multinucleated giant cells Mesenchyme
Papillary	+	+	−	−	±	M	−	+	−	−	Papillae Tall columnar cells Hemosiderin macrophages
Secretory	−	±	±	+	+	M	+	−	−	±	Demarcated vacuolated cells
Tubular	−	−	+	+	+	M	−	−	−	−	Tubules

* Isolated cells in all.

† Large, >30 μm; medium, 15–30 μm; small, <15 μm.

sisting of fibrosarcomatous, liposarcomatous, myxosarcomatous, or rhabdomyosar-comatous elements.[71] Only the mesenchymal elements metastasize.

Recurrence is probably due to inadequate excision because of grossly inapparent, small neoplastic projections. Hematogenously spread tumors most commonly are found in the lung, followed by the bones, heart, and brain.[45] Regional lymph nodes are infrequently involved; axillary nodes may be enlarged because of inflammation secondary to necrotic breast tumor.[5] From the Armed Forces Institute of Pathology files, 80 percent of 94 patients had recurrences, generally within 2 years, and 17 percent died of metastatic disease within 6 years. All fatal tumors were at least 4.0 cm in diameter and demonstrated three or more mitoses per 10 high-power fields.[71]

The tumor is usually estrogen receptor negative but strongly positive for proges-terone receptors.[81] Carcinoembryonic antigen (CEA) positivity in the tumorous epithelium may predict recurrence.[2] Treatment consists of generous lumpectomy in benign cases, while malignant forms are treated by simple mastectomy.

ABC: Morphologically Benign

The aspirate resembles that from a fibroadenoma. The cell-rich ABC consists of tissue fragments, monolayered sheets, and naked nuclei. There are numerous cell-dense fronds with finger-like projections, as well as sheets composed of as many as 500 or as few as 10 cells. Unlike the ABC from fibroadenoma, the tissue fragments may be edematous with a fibromyxomatous pattern, and there may be fragments of myxoid stroma.

The constituents of these units are cohesive, well-polarized, uniform small cells with oval nuclei displaying finely granular chromatin and prominent nucleoli. The abundant naked, bipolar or oval nuclei have similar characteristics. Benign multinu-cleated giant cells, foam cells, and histiocytes may be interspersed (Fig. 7.14).

Can benign cystosarcoma be differentiated from fibroadenoma by ABC? Some-times the cellular specimens are indistinguishable, with large, cohesive cellular clus-ters and numerous naked nuclei. Features especially associated with cystosarcoma are cell richness with both epithelial fronds and fibromyxoid tissue fragments, as well as the special clinical presentation of a large, rapidly growing mass in a peri- or postmenopausal woman. Simi et al.[93] observed foam cells and multinucleated giant cells with no evidence of apocrine cells in four of five cases of cystosarcoma, whereas in 20 fibroadenomas, apocrine cells were plentiful in 75 percent of the cases while rare giant cells were present in only 10 percent. Silverman et al.[92] interpreted three of six benign cystosarcomas correctly; one was interpreted as fibroadenoma and two carcinoma.

ABC: Morphologically Malignant

Cardozo[9] was the first to point out the biphasic pattern of the ABC, the dual popu-lations characterizing the tumor. Both sarcomatous and epithelial components can be either well differentiated or poorly differentiated. Although they are solid le-sions, cystic specimens have been described.[96]

The cell-rich aspirate is composed of many isolated sarcomatous cells, a few small, dyshesive epithelial groups, and naked nuclei. There may also be a few fronds distinguishing the neoplasm from other sarcomas. The predominant spindle cells,

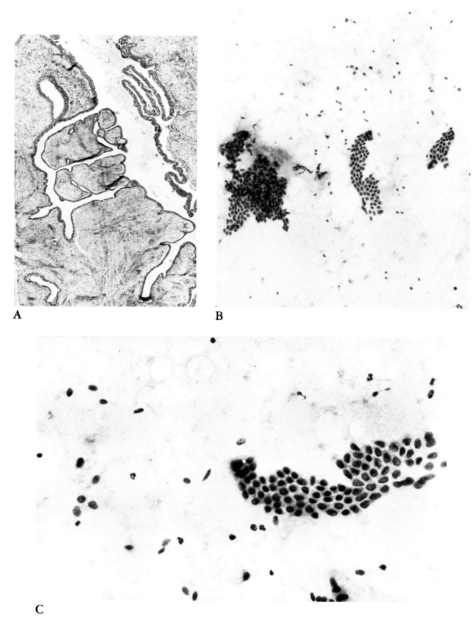

C

Fig. 7.14. Cystosarcoma phyllodes, benign. **A.** Tissue section. Note the bulky nodules projecting into the cystic space. Hematoxylin and eosin preparation (×30). **B.** ABC. Note the fronds and naked nuclei, similar to those of fibroadenoma. Papanicolaou preparation (×125). **C.** ABC, higher magnification. Note the edematous sheet. Papanicolaou preparation (×300).

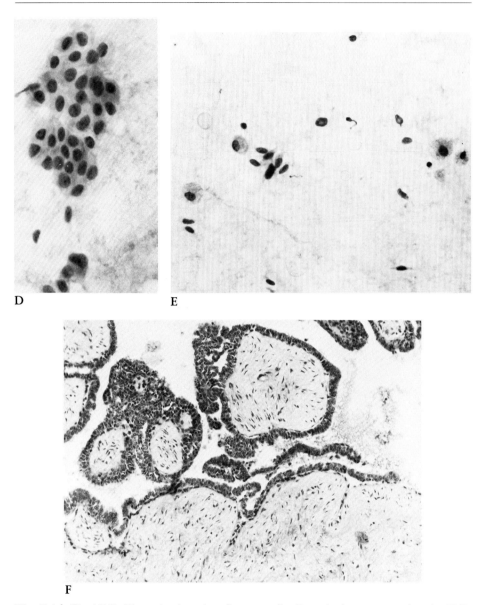

Fig. 7.14. **D.** ABC. Note the loosely adherent cells. Papanicolaou preparation (×500).
E. ABC. Note the naked nuclei and foam cells. Papanicolaou preparation (×300). **F.** Tissue
section. Hematoxylin and eosin preparation (×125).

ranging from 15 to 35 μm in length, have scant, pale cytoplasm and central, single or multiple, irregular nuclei with some macronucleoli. The relatively little epithelium may consist of bland cuboidal or columnar cells with eccentric nuclei and ill-defined cytoplasm or occasional bizarre cells with three or four pleomorphic nuclei. Round, oval, or elongated naked nuclei, measuring 6 to 22 μm, with irregular membranes, finely or coarsely granular chromatin, and prominent nucleoli, may be seen (Fig. 7.15).

The major interpretative trap associated with this neoplasm is the same with ABC as with histologic sections: the lack of specific features indicative of biological behavior. False-positive interpretation is not rare.[29,92] Therefore, decision making cannot be based on the ABC but only on tissue, including multiple sections from the margins.

OTHER SARCOMAS

These tumors, exclusive of cystosarcoma, constitute less than 0.2 percent of all malignant breast neoplasms. Due to their rarity, it is not surprising that there are few examples in the cytologic literature. Case descriptions include rhabdomyosarcoma,[101] stromal sarcoma[84] chloroma,[79] primary osteogenic sarcoma[68] and angiosarcoma.[64,75] From the 1,745 malignant breast tumors examined by ABC at the Curie Institute,[107] the incidence of sarcoma was 0.2 percent, and from our institution it was 0.15 percent.

Malignant fibrous histiocytomas, generally found in the lower extremities of

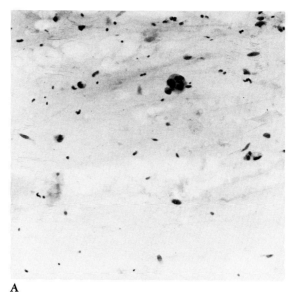

A

Fig. 7.15. Cytosarcoma phyllodes, malignant. A. ABC. Note the cell-rich specimen with isolated, pleomorphic cells. Papanicolaou preparation (×125).

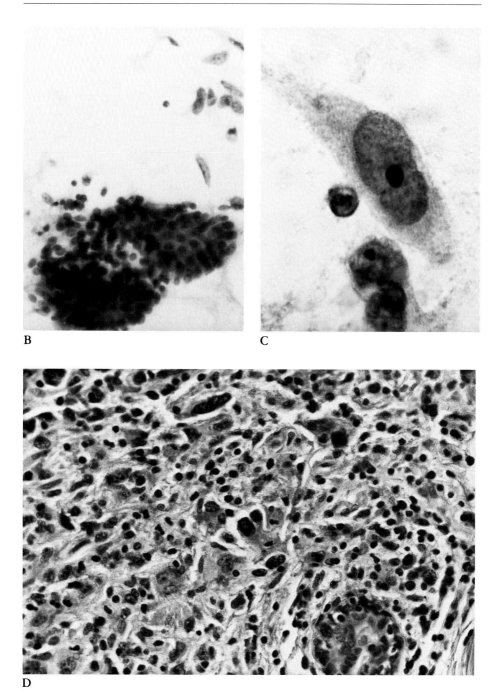

B

C

D

Fig. 7.15. **B.** ABC. Note the frond. Papanicolaou preparation (× 300). **C.** ABC. Note the bizarre isolated cell. Papanicolaou preparation (× 1250). **D.** Tissue section. Hematoxylin and eosin preparation (× 300).

elderly men, are very unusual in the breast. Radiation may be a causative factor; in one review, three of eight women with the neoplasm had been irradiated for breast carcinoma.[58] The somewhat circumscribed neoplasms have a variable histologic appearance, most commonly the pleomorphic storiform (basket-weave) pattern. The ABC findings from the five cases cited in the literature[58,63,92] generally were cell rich, consisting of many bizarre isolated cells with some multinucleation. Some of the tumor cells had phagocytized debris and red blood cells. In two cases, tissue fragments suggested a storiform pattern, but in none were there Touton giant cells.

The sarcomas examined by ABC in our institution included a low-grade leiomyosarcoma and a fibrosarcoma. The former appeared in an 84-year-old man as a periareolar mass. The cellular ABC consisted of dyshesive tissue fragments and isolated spindle cells. The spindle cells, measuring up to 50 μm, had a modest amount of indistinctly delineated cytoplasm with single or multiple nuclei. The nuclei were somewhat variable in shape, with finely granular chromatin and prominent nucleoli (Fig. 7.16).

From our second patient, a 54-year-old woman with fibrosarcoma, the specimen consisted of 50 cc of chocolate-colored fluid, and there was a residual mass. The ABC was composed of scattered, chiefly isolated, spindled, bizarre cells in a background of blood and debris. The tumor cells, ranging from 15 to 30 μm in length, had ill-defined, wispy cytoplasm and irregular, cigar-shaped nuclei with a few macronucleoli (Fig. 7.17).

SECONDARY NEOPLASMS

Pathology

Metastases to the breast have an incidence of 0.13 to 0.45 percent, excluding contralateral mammary carcinoma.[37,87] Lung and prostate are the chief sites of origin,[86] but malignant melanoma, uterine carcinoma, carcinoid, leukemia, and sarcoma all have been described, occasionally arising from an occult tumor.[37,88] The well-demarcated metastases may be as large as 15 cm, and generally are neither necrotic nor calcified. All studies emphasize the problem of differentiating an extramammary from a primary breast neoplasm, particularly by mammography and frozen section.[74,89]

ABC

Correct interpretation of metastatic malignant cells procured by NAB of the breast depends on two factors: clinical findings and recognition of alien cells. The cells usually can be identified as malignant because they demonstrate all the malignant criteria. Awareness that these are foreign cells, however, depends upon a thorough understanding of the ABC from primary breast neoplasms, their pattern, cell size, and cytoplasmic and nuclear detail.

The importance of the team approach is self-evident. There is no substitute for the clinical history. Knowledge of the site of needle penetration also may be crucial (e.g., whether lymphoid cells are from the breast or from the axillary nodes). Addi-

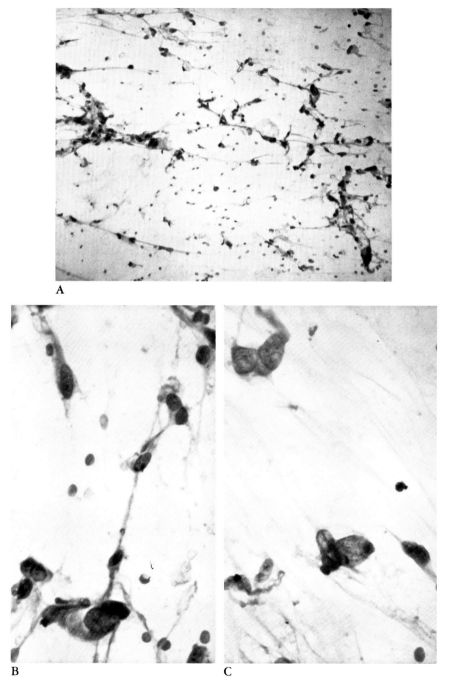

Fig. 7.16. Leiomyosarcoma in the male breast. **A.** ABC. Note the cellularity with dyshesive fragments and isolated cells. Papanicolaou preparation (×125). **B,C.** ABC. Note the nuclei with variable shapes and bland chromatin. Papanicolaou preparations (×500).

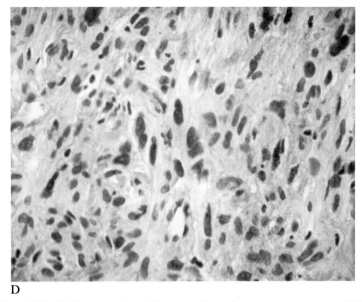

D

Fig. 7.16. D. Tissue section. Hematoxylin and eosin preparation (×300).

tionally, grittiness from needle contact with calcified particles is rare in secondary neoplasms.

The pattern of the ABC requires analysis. Many have a tumor diathesis. Melanoma, neuroendocrine tumor, and hepatocellular carcinoma each have distinctive characteristics.[47] Acini of the metastatic adenocarcinoma must be distinguished from dyshesive clusters of the infiltrating ductal carcinoma and from syncytia of the medullary carcinoma. Papillae of metastatic thyroid, ovarian, or endometrial carcinoma must be differentiated from those of mammary papillary carcinoma. A plethora of bizarre single cells from malignant melanoma, metastatic squamous carcinoma, or transitional cell carcinoma must be differentiated from those of medullary carcinoma.

Evaluation of naked nuclei can prove diagnostic. The cells of lymphoma and small cell carcinoma must be separated from the bare nuclei of fibroadenoma and carcinoma, including the medullary, apocrine, and papillary carcinomas. We misinterpreted as lymphoma the small cells from an occult pulmonary oat cell carcinoma, overlooking necrosis as well as the molding and oat shape of some of the cells. By contrast, cells from lymphoma consist of large and small lymphocytes with macronucleoli and mitoses and without phagocytosis[52] (Fig. 7.18; Table 7.5).

The individual cells must be scrutinized for size, nuclear alterations, and cytoplasmic inclusions. Size may provide an important clue; with the exception of medullary carcinoma, large tumor cells are unusual in primary breast carcinoma. Nuclear examination can be revealing; pleomorphism, nuclear clear zones, and bizarre macronucleoli are rare in primary neoplasms. Cytoplasmic inspection can be most helpful. Cytoplasmic mucin in signet-ring, secretory, and adenoid cystic carcinomas is sparse, by contrast to the abundance characteristic of some metastatic adenocarcinomas. Pigment can be diagnostic, and melanin is differentiated from hemosiderin by the iron and Fontana-Masson stains.[85] Granules from metastatic carcinoids may

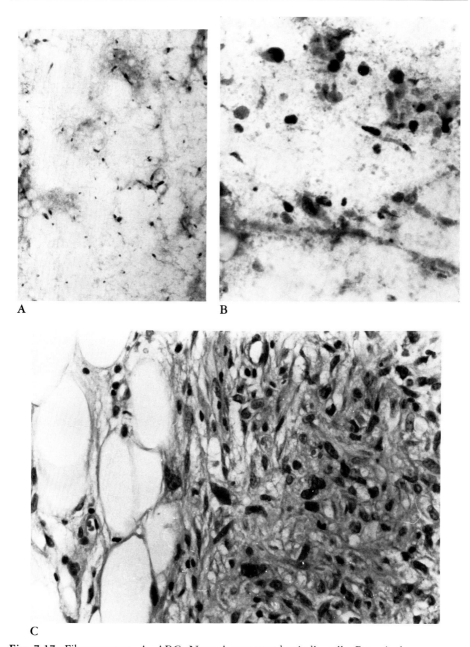

A   B

C

Fig. 7.17. Fibrosarcoma. **A.** ABC. Note the scattered spindle cells. Papanicolaou preparation (×125). **B.** ABC. Note the cells with cigar-shaped nuclei and tumor diathesis. Papanicolaou preparation (×300). **C.** Tissue section. Hematoxylin and eosin preparation (×300).

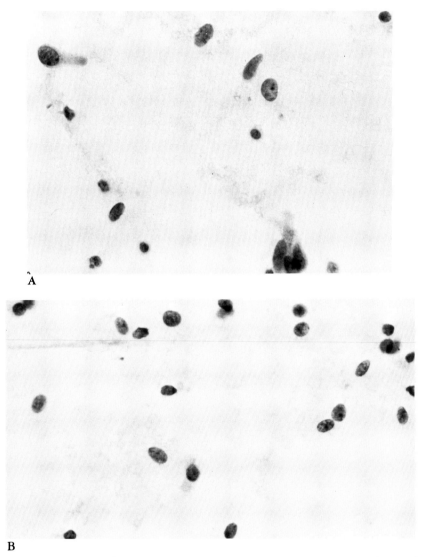

A

B

Fig. 7.18. Contrasting naked nuclei, ABC. **A.** Papillary carcinoma. Note the elongated and oval nuclei. Papanicolaou preparation ($\times 500$). **B.** Fibroadenoma. Note the bipolar and oval naked nuclei. Papanicolaou preparation ($\times 500$).

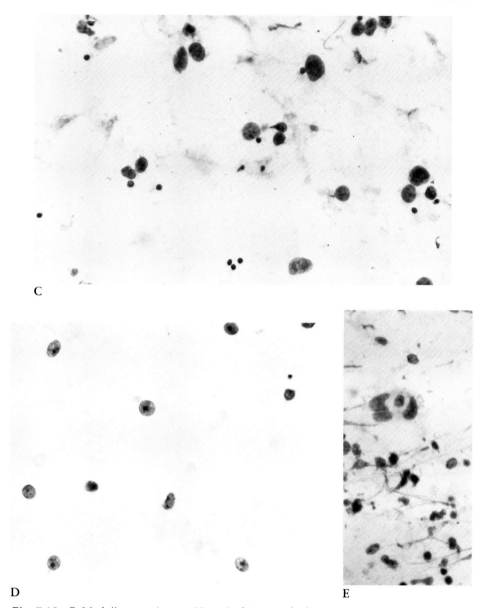

C

D   E

Fig. 7.18. C. Medullary carcinoma. Note the bizarre naked nuclei. Papanicolaou preparation (×500). D. Lactating adenoma. Note the vesicular, round naked nuclei with macronucleoli. Papanicolaou preparation (×500). E. Oat cell carcinoma. Note molding and necrotic debris. Papanicolaou preparation (×500).

TABLE 7.5. Naked Nuclei*; Comparative Cytomorphology

Histology	Shape	Size (μm)	Special Features
Fibroadenoma	Bipolar	6–7	Fronds
	Round		
	Spindled		
Carcinomas			
Adenoid cystic	Round	6–8	Mucoid cores
Apocrine	Round	6–8	Apocrine cells
Medullary	Bizarre	12–15	Pleomorphic cells
			Lymphocytes
Papillary	Elongated	6–15	Papillae
Lymphoma	Round	4–8	Macronucleoli
Small-cell carcinoma	Round	10–15	Molding
	Oat		Necrosis

*All lesions may demonstrate some anisonucleosis and occasional macronucleoli.

be identified by the Grimelius stain.[4] All these histochemical as well as immunocytochemical reactions can provide critical diagnostic information (see Chapter 11).

Metastatic melanoma has been specifically diagnosed from the ABC by us and others even without pigmentation.[55,91,104] The isolated cells, with a scant or abundant cytoplasm, are divisible into two or three distinct populations: small, 10–12 μm; moderate, 15–20 μm; and giant size. Plasmacytoid cells, multinucleation, nuclei with intranuclear cytoplasmic invaginations, and eosinophilic macronucleoli are frequent[49] (Fig. 7.19).

Specimens from other metastases to the breast may be relatively distinctive. The cell-rich ABC from metastatic prostatic carcinoma consists of isolated cells and some small, dyshesive groups of cells with ill-defined cytoplasm and vesicular nuclei with thickened membranes, anisonucleosis, and macronucleoli. The cells demonstrate positivity to prostatic-specific antigen or prostatic acid phosphatase by the immunoperoxidase technique applied directly to the Papanicolaou-stained slide[44] (see Plate 1.4). The ABC from metastatic endometrial carcinoma, seen by us and others,[91,105] has a pattern of cell balls, large papillary groups with peripheral columnar cells, and dyshesive acini in a necrotic diathesis. The relatively uniform cells, measuring up to 20 μm, have a scant, indistinctly delineated cytoplasm and large nuclei; macronucleoli are unusual (Fig. 7.20). From metastatic colonic carcinoma, we have identified distinctive spear-shaped groups and isolated malignant cells; tall columnar cells may have eosinophilic macronucleoli (Fig. 7.21). From metastatic carcinoid, the cell-rich ABC is distinguished by monolayered dyshesive groups, small single cells, vesicular naked nuclei, and Grimelius-positive cytoplasmic granules.[57,94] Metastases from cervical squamous carcinoma,[61] renal cell carcinoma,[73] and mycosis fungoides[89] have been described. Silverman et al.[91] correctly interpreted the ABC from 18 breast metastases: 4 pulmonary carcinomas; 5 from the female genital tract; 3 lymphoreticular malignancies; 2 melanomas; and 1 neuroblastoma, bladder carcinoma, hepatocellular carcinoma, and prostatic carcinoma.

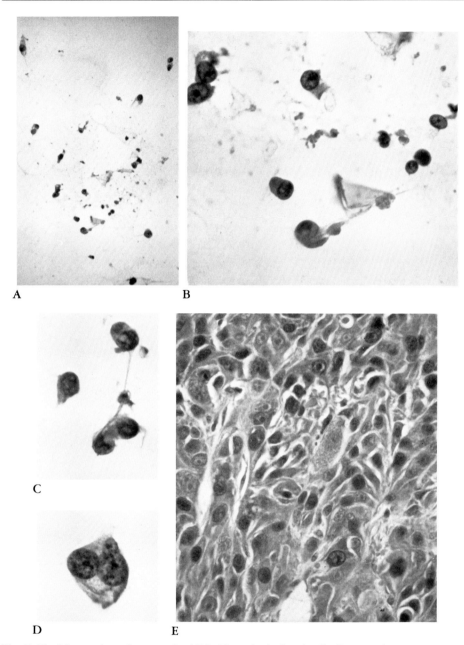

Fig. 7.19. Metastatic melanoma. **A.** ABC. Note the isolated cells. Papanicolaou preparation (×125). **B.** ABC. Note the plasmacytoid cells. Papanicolaou preparation (×300). **C.** ABC. Note nuclear clear zones. Papanicolaou preparation (×300). **D.** ABC. Note the multinucleation and macronucleoli. Papanicolaou preparation (×500). **E.** Tissue section. Hematoxylin and eosin preparation (×300). (Courtesy of Denise Hidvegi, M.D., Northwestern University, Chicago.)

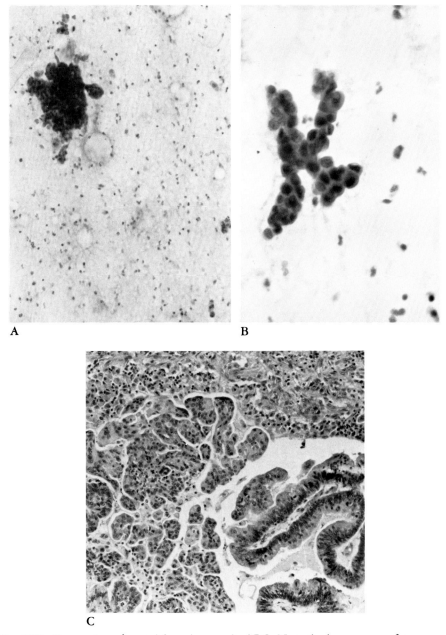

A

B

C

Fig. 7.20. Metastatic endometrial carcinoma. **A.** ABC. Note the large group of tumor cells and necrotic diathesis. Papanicolaou preparation ($\times$125). **B.** ABC. Note the papilla with relatively uniform cells with a cytoplasmic rim. Papanicolaou preparation ($\times$300). **C.** Tissue section. Hematoxylin and eosin preparation ($\times$125).

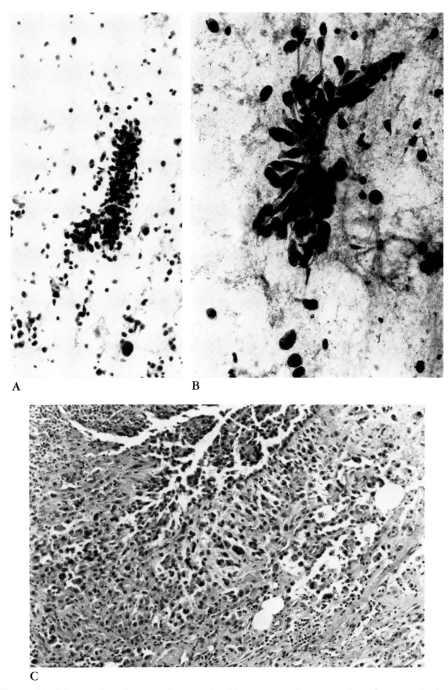

Fig. 7.21. Metastatic colon carcinoma. **A.** ABC. Note the spear-shaped group, isolated tumor cells, and tumor diathesis. Papanicolaou preparation (×125). **B.** ABC. Note the acinus composed of tall columnar cells. Papanicolaou preparation (×500). **C.** Tissue section. Hematoxylin and eosin preparation (×125).

CARCINOMA IN MEN

Pathology

The incidence of male mammary malignant tumors varies from 0.4 to 1.5 percent[18] and has remained constant for several decades.[22] It constitutes about 0.7 percent of the 135,900 anticipated yearly cases in the United States.[90] Although the median age of onset is 60, it has been reported from age 5 to 93, with bilaterality in 1.4 percent of the cases.[18] Clinically, the most common finding is a painless periareolar mass, sometimes accompanied by a sanguineous nipple discharge.[18] It may be mistaken for gynecomastia, and in fact, there may be an association between the two lesions.[62] Familial history may be a risk factor,[59] and hormone therapy for prostatic carcinoma may play a role in its development.[18]

The infiltrating ductal carcinoma is the usual carcinoma in men, but mucinous, medullary, papillary, and intraductal carcinomas, as well as Paget's disease, inflammatory carcinoma, and cystosarcoma, are seen.[18,33,40,62] Small-cell carcinoma with features of infiltrating lobular carcinoma, but lacking the intraductal component, also has been reported.[33]

Initially, it was believed that carcinomas were more virulent in men than in women, but later reports indicate a similar survival.[95] There seems to be a longer period of development prior to seeking medical attention; in one group, half of the patients had positive nodes at the initial examination.[18] The tumors are frequently estrogen receptor positive, and many are tamoxifen sensitive. Combination chemotherapy also gives a response rate similar to that of women with breast carcinoma.[6]

ABC

Studies concerning the cytomorphology of male breast carcinoma are rare. Our material consists of 13 cases: 9 infiltrating ductal carcinomas, a mucinous carcinoma, a leiomyosarcoma, and metastatic carcinoma from the prostate and colon (Figs. 7.22, 7.23; see Plate 1.4; the sections on "Other Sarcomas" and "Secondary Neoplasms" in this chapter; and Chapter 6 for the ABC). In one argyrophilic carcinoma, the characteristic tumor cells reacted positively to estrogen receptor.[94]

CYSTIC CARCINOMA

Pathology

Carcinomas associated with cysts are unusual lesions. The incidence was 0.5 percent among 9,000 mastectomy specimens removed for malignant tumor.[32] These included 33 papillary carcinomas, 10 comedo carcinomas, 3 in-situ lobular carcinomas, and 12 other types. The cysts measured 1.0 to 10.0 cm in diameter; most were solitary, of which four were multiloculated. Benign cysts were invaded by tumor in a third of the cases, and the three in-situ carcinomas were discovered serendipitously. Czernobilsky[20] reported a similar incidence (0.56 percent), distinguishing between true intracystic carcinoma, usually papillary, and cystic-type neoplasms, i.e., solid tumors infiltrating a benign cyst or with areas of cystic necrosis. In our experience, the tumor most likely to show cystic degeneration is medullary carcinoma.[41]

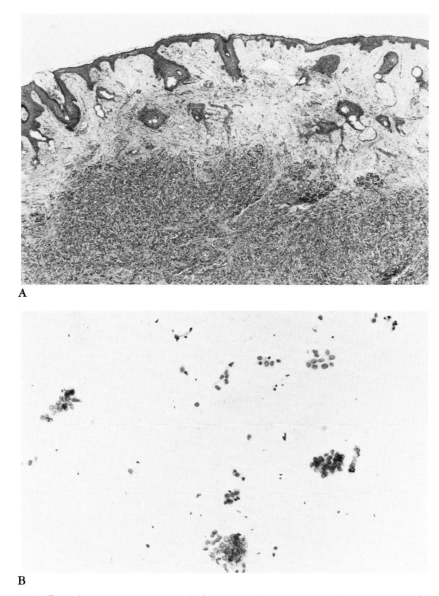

A

B

Fig. 7.22. Ductal carcinoma in the male breast. **A.** Tissue section. Hematoxylin and eosin preparation (×30). **B.** ABC. Note the cell richness with dyshesive clusters of monomorphic cells. Papanicolaou preparation (×125).

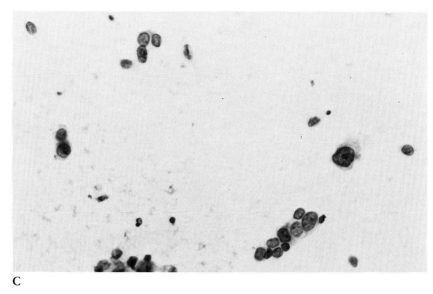

C

Fig. 7.22. C. ABC. Note the dyshesive clusters of moderate-sized cells showing all the criteria of malignancy. Papanicolaou preparation (×300).

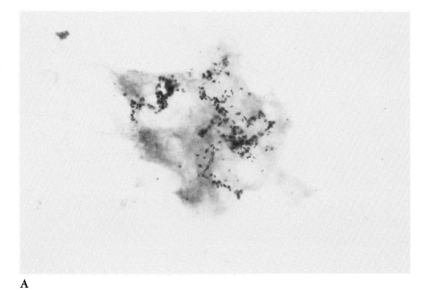

A

Fig. 7.23. Mucinous carcinoma in the male breast. **A.** ABC. Note the dyshesive clusters and isolated cells within mucin. Papanicolaou preparation (×125).

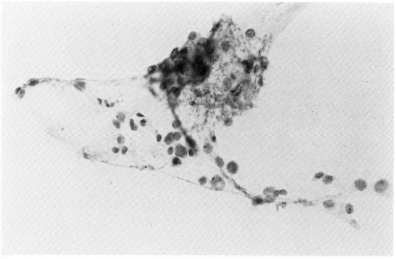

B

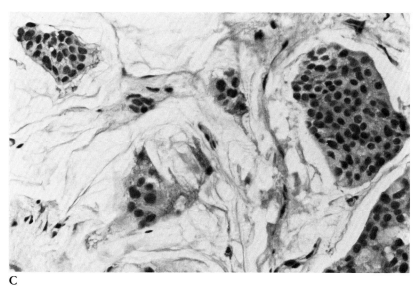

C

Fig. 7.23. B. ABC. Note the cell ball and isolated cells within mucinous strands. Papanicolaou preparation (×300). **C.** Tissue section. Hematoxylin and eosin preparation (×300).

ABC

In 1933 Stewart[97] stated that NAB was indicated "to differentiate the thick-walled, deep-seated abscess or cyst from carcinoma." Papanicolaou et al.[76] wrote that the "cyst aspirate smear appears to be a particularly valuable tool for differentiating between benign and malignant breast cysts." McSwain et al.[67] reported an incidence of 1.7 percent of 595 cyst fluids associated with carcinoma, and Abramson[1] reported an incidence of 0.8 percent among 1,275 cysts; in the latter study, 16 patients with apparent cysts were found to have solid tumors by NAB. Many reports, however, indicate that examination of fluids is unnecessary, since the tumors can all be detected by bloody taps and incompletely collapsed cysts or ones that refill.[16,28] Ciatto et al.,[15] after their experience with 6,782 cystic lesions, concluded that microscopic study should be limited to hemorrhagic fluid.

In our experience, while 22 percent of our 13,000 aspirates were from cysts, only 1 percent of the fluid specimens contained tumor cells, and most carcinomas were suspected clinically. Interestingly, in 0.2 percent, however, malignant cells were retrieved from straw-colored fluid, and no mass remained. The majority of our "malignant" fluids were derived from solid tumors with cystic necrosis, including five medullary carcinomas (see the section on "Medullary Carcinoma" in Chapter 6), a metaplastic carcinoma, a fibrosarcoma, and several ductal and comedo carcinomas.[41,46] Two intracystic papillary carcinomas were diagnosed from hemorrhagic fluid specimens[50] (see Figs. 6.14, 6.15, 7.9). In one case, the tumor cells originated in an in-situ lobular carcinoma adjacent to a benign cyst (see Fig 12.3 and Tables 7.1 and 7.3).

Examination of fluid aspirates can be difficult. False-positive results are due to misinterpretation of cells from intraductal papillomas and apocrine cysts[48] (see the section on "Apocrine Cysts" in Chapter 4 and the section on "Papillomas" in Chapter 5). False-negative interpretation occurs because of dilution, shrinkage, and degeneration of malignant cells; tumor cells hidden by neutrophils, necrotic debris, or blood; or nonsampling of a residual mass. Preparations such as membrane filtration, cytocentrifugation, or paraffin blocks, rather than direct smears, are useful for concentration and visualization of the tumor cells, while the team approach is essential for evaluation of the clinical findings (see Fig. 7.9 and Chapter 2).

In summary, many contend that cyst fluid should be examined only if it is hemorrhagic or collected from a residual or recurrent mass. Our findings indicate, however, that a few carcinomas (<1 percent) would be undetected. What, therefore, should be the philosophy of those performing the NAB: to examine or not to examine the fluids? Resolution of the problem will be guided by legal suits, insurance schemes, spiraling medical costs, and the individual patient. (see the section on "The Surgeon and NAB" in Chapter 8).

INFLAMMATORY CARCINOMA

The rapidly lethal inflammatory carcinoma derives its name from its clinical presentation, with the cardinal signs of inflammation. The breast is hyperemic, reddened, painful, and edematous, giving the skin its peau d'orange appearance. Histologically, the carcinoma is characterized not by specific type of tumor but rather by tumorous

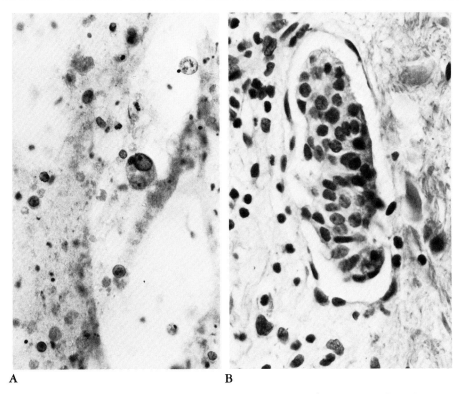

A   B

Fig. 7.24. Inflammatory carcinoma. **A.** ABC. Note the scattered malignant cells in the tumor diathesis. Papanicolaou preparation (×300). **B.** Tissue section. Note the tumor cells in the lymphatic vessel. Hematoxylin and eosin preparation (×300).

invasion of the dermal and epidermal lymphatics. In a series of 64 patients with unilateral inflammatory breast carcinoma constituting 6 percent of all breast carcinomas, the average age was 49, half of the patients being in their reproductive years; median survival was 23 months.[13]

Since inflammatory carcinoma and mastitis resemble each other, NAB is critical for their distinction. The ABC is characteristic of a malignant tumor: many cells with nuclear membrane irregularity, anisonucleosis, and macronucleoli in a diathesis of debris, inflammation, and blood. From a series of seven patients ultimately diagnosed as having inflammatory carcinoma, the ABC from six was interpreted as positive, and from one, suggestive of carcinoma.[46] One 60-year-old woman presented with localized inflammation; the aspiration biopsy, performed chiefly for culture of the probable abscess, revealed malignant cells compatible with inflammatory carcinoma (Fig. 7.24).

REFERENCES

1. Abramson DJ: A clinical evaluation of aspiration of cysts of the breast. *Surg Gynecol Obstet* 139:531–537, 1974.

2. Alberti O Jr, Brentani MM, Goes JCS, et al: Carcinoembryonic antigen; a possible predictor of recurrence in cystosarcoma phyllodes. *Cancer* 57:1042–1045, 1986.

3. d'Amore ESG, Maisto L, Gatteschi MB, Toma S, Canavese G: Secretory carcinoma of the breast; report of a case with fine needle aspiration biopsy. *Acta Cytol* 30:309–312, 1986.

4. Ascoli V, Newman GA, Kline TS: Grimelius stain for cytodiagnosis of carcinoid tumor. *Diagn Cytopathol* 2:157–159, 1986.

5. Azzopardi JG: *Problems in Breast Pathology.* Philadelphia, WB Saunders Co, 1979.

6. Bezwoda WR, Hesdorffer C, Dansey R, et al: Breast cancer in men; clinical features, hormone receptor status, and response to therapy. *Cancer* 60:1337–1340, 1987.

7. Boccato P, Briani G, d'Atri C, et al: Spindle cell and cartilaginous metaplasia in a breast carcinoma with osteoclastlike stromal cells; a difficult fine needle aspiration diagnosis. *Acta Cytol* 32:75–78, 1988.

8. Bondeson L: Aspiration cytology of breast carcinoma with multinucleated reactive stromal giant cells. *Acta Cytol* 28:313–316, 1984.

9. Cardozo PL: *Atlas of Clinical Cytology.* Targa b.v.'s Hertogenbosch, the Netherlands, 1973.

10. Carstens PHB, Greenberg RA, Francis D, Lyon H: Tubular carcinoma of the breast; a long term follow-up. *Histopathology* 9:271–280, 1985.

11. Carter D, Orr SL, Merino MJ; Intracystic papillary carcinoma of the breast; after mastectomy, radiotherapy, or excisional biopsy alone. *Cancer* 52:14–19, 1983.

12. Cavanzo FJ, Taylor HB: Adenoid cystic carcinoma of the breast; an analysis of 21 cases. *Cancer* 24:740–745, 1969.

13. Chevallier B, Asselain B, Kunlin A, et al: Inflammatory breast cancer; determination of prognostic factors by univariate and multivariate analysis. *Cancer* 60:897–902, 1987.

14. Chilosi M, Bonetti F, Menestrina F, Lestani M: Breast carcinoma with stromal multinucleated giant cells. *J Pathol* 152:55–56, 1987.

15. Ciatto S, Cariaggi P, Bularesi P: The value of routine cytologic examination of breast cyst fluids. *Acta Cytol* 31:301–304, 1987.

16. Cowen PN, Benson EA: Cytological study of fluid from breast cysts. *Br J Surg* 66:209–211, 1979.

17. Craig JP: Secretory carcinoma of the breast in an adult; correlation of aspiration cytology and histology on the biopsy specimen. *Acta Cytol* 29:589–592, 1985.

18. Crichlow RW: Carcinoma of the male breast. *Surg Gynecol Obstet* 134:1011–1019, 1972.

19. Cubilla AL, Woodruff JM: Primary carcinoid tumor of the breast: A report of eight patients. *Am J Surg Pathol* 1:283–292, 1977.

20. Czernobilsky B: Intracystic carcinoma of the female breast. *Surg Gynecol Obstet* 124:93–98, 1967.

21. DeLellis RA, Dayal Y, Wolfe HJ: Carcinoid tumors; changing concepts and new perspectives. *Am J Surg Pathol* 8:295–299, 1984.

22. Devesa SS, Silverman DT, Young JL Jr, et al: Cancer incidence and mortality trends among whites in the United States, 1947–1984. *JNCI* 79:701–770, 1987.

23. Duggan MA, Young GK, Hwang WS: Fine-needle aspiration of an apocrine breast carcinoma with multivacuolated, lipid-rich, giant cells. *Diagn Cytopathol* 4:62–66, 1988.

24. Fisher ER, Alka S, Palekar AS, NSABP Collaborators: Solid and mucinous varieties of so-called mammary carcinoid tumors. *Am J Clin Pathol* 72:909–916, 1979.

25. Fisher ER, Gregorio RM, Palekar AS, Paulson JD: Mucoepidermoid and squamous cell carcinomas of breast with reference to squamous metaplasia and giant cell tumors. *Am J Surg Pathol* 7:15–27, 1983.

26. Fisher ER, Palekar AS, Redmond C, Barton B, Fisher B: Pathologic findings from the National Surgical Adjuvant Breast Project (Protocol No. 4); VI. invasive papillary cancer. *Am J Clin Pathol* 73:313–321, 1980.

27. Fisher ER, Tavares J, Bulatao IS, et al: Glycogen-rich, clear cell breast cancer: With comments concerning other clear cell variants. *Hum Pathol* 16:1085–1090, 1985.

28. Forrest APM, Kirkpatrick JR, Roberts MM: Needle aspiration of breast cysts. *Br Med J* 3:30–31, 1975.

29. Frable WJ: Needle aspiration of the breast. *Cancer* 53:671–676, 1984.

30. Frable WJ, Kay S: Carcinoma of the breast; histologic and clinical features of apocrine tumors. *Cancer* 21:756–763, 1968.

31. Gal R, Gukovsky-Oren S, Lehman JM, Schwartz P, Kessler E: Cytodiagnosis of a spindle-cell tumor of the breast using antisera to epithelial membrane antigen. *Acta Cytol* 31:317–321, 1987.

32. Gatchell FG, Dockerty MB, Clagett OT: Intracystic carcinoma of the breast. *Surg Gynecol Obstet* 106:347–352, 1958.

33. Giffler RF, Kay S: Small-cell carcinoma of the male mammary breast; a tumor resembling infiltrating lobular carcinoma. *Am J Clin Pathol* 66:715–721, 1976.

34. Gompel C, Van Kerkem C: The breast, in Silverberg SG (ed): *Principles and Practice of Surgical Pathology,* Vol. 1. New York, John Wiley & Sons, Inc 1983, pp 245–295.

35. Gupta RK, Wakefield SJ, Holloway LJ, Simpson JS: Immunocytochemical and ultra-structural study of the rare osteoclast-type carcinoma of the breast in a fine needle aspirate. *Acta Cytol* 32:79–82, 1988.

36. Hajdu SI, Espinosa MH, Robbins GF: Recurrent cystosarcoma phyllodes. *Cancer* 38:1402–1406, 1976.

37. Hajdu SI, Urban JA: Cancer metastatic to the breast. *Cancer* 29:1691–1696, 1972.

38. Hamperl H: Das sogenannte Schweissdrusen-carcinom der Mamma; eine Ubersicht. *Z Krebsforsch* 88:105–119, 1977.

39. Hasleton PS, Misch KA, Vasudev KS, George D: Squamous carcinoma of the breast. *J Clin Pathol* 31:116–124, 1978.

40. Heller KS, Rosen PP, Schottenfeld D, Ashikari R, Kinne DW: Male breast cancer; a clinicopathologic study of 97 cases. *Ann Surg* 188:60–65, 1978.

41. Howell LP, Kline TS: Medullary carcinoma of the breast: An unusual cytologic finding in cyst fluid aspirates. *Cancer* in press.

42. Hsui J-G, Hawkins AG, d'Amato NA, Mullen JT: A case of pure primary squamous carcinoma of the breast diagnosed by fine needle aspiration biopsy. *Acta Cytol* 29:650–651, 1985.

43. Hull MT, Warfel KA: Glycogen-rich clear cell carcinomas of the breast; a clinico-pathologic and ultrastructural study. *Am J Surg Pathol* 10:553–559, 1986.

44. Keshgegian AA, Kline TS: Immunoperoxidase demonstration of prostatic acid phosphatase in aspiration biopsy cytology (ABC). *Am J Clin Pathol* 82:586–589, 1984.

45. Kessinger A, Foley JF, Lemon HM, Miller DD: Metastatic cystosarcoma phyllodes: A case report and review of the literature. *J Surg Oncol* 4:131–147, 1972.

46. Kline TS: Breast lesions; diagnosis by fine-needle aspiration biopsy. *Am J Diagn Gynecol Obstet* 1:11–16, 1979.

47. Kline TS: *Handbook of Fine Needle Aspiration Biopsy Cytology*, ed 2. New York, Churchill Livingstone, 1988.

48. Kline TS: Masquerades of malignancy: A review of 4241 aspirates from the breast. *Acta Cytol* 25:263–266, 1981.

49. Kline TS, Kannan V: Aspiration biopsy cytology and melanoma. *Am J Clin Pathol* 77:597–601, 1983.

50. Kline TS, Kannan V: Papillary carcinoma of the breast; a cytomorphologic analysis. *Arch Pathol Lab Med* 110:189–191, 1986.

51. Kline TS, Kannan V, Kline IK: Appraisal and cytomorphologic analysis of common carcinomas of the breast. *Diagn Cytopathol* 1:188–193, 1985.

52. Kline TS, Kannan V, Kline IK: Lymphadenopathy and aspiration biopsy cytology; review of 376 superficial nodes. *Cancer* 54:1076–1081, 1984.

53. Kline TS, Kline IK: Metaplastic carcinoma of the breast—diagnosis by ABC; report of two cases and literature review. *Diagn Cytopathol* in press.

54. Koss LG, Brannan CD, Ashikari R: Histologic and ultrastructural features of adenoid cystic carcinoma of the breast. *Cancer* 26:1271–1279, 1970.

55. Koss LG, Woyke S, Olszewski W: *Aspiration Biopsy: Cytologic Interpretation and Histologic Bases*. New York, Igaku-Shoin, 1984.

56. Kraus FT, Neubecker RD: The differential diagnosis of papillary tumors of the breast. *Cancer* 15:444–455, 1962.

57. Landon G, Sneige N, Ordonez NG, Mackay B: Carcinoid metastatic to breast diagnosed by fine-needle aspiration biopsy. *Diagn Cytopathol* 3:230–233, 1987.

58. Langham MR, Mills AS, DeMay RM, et al: Malignant fibrous histiocytoma of the breast; a case report and review of the literature. *Cancer* 54:558–563, 1984.

59. LaRaja RD, Pagnozzi JA, Rothenberg RE, et al: Carcinoma of the breast in three siblings. *Cancer* 55:2709–2711, 1985.

60. Lazarevic B, Rodgers JB: Aspiration cytology of carcinoid tumor of the breast; a case report. *Acta Cytol* 27:329–333, 1983.

61. Leiman G: Squamous carcinoma of the breast: Diagnosis by aspiration cytology. *Acta Cytol* 26:201–209, 1982.

62. Liechty RD, Davis J, Gleysteen J: Cancer of the male breast; forty cases. *Cancer* 20:1617–1624, 1967.

63. Luzzatto R, Grossmann S, Scholl JG, Recktenvald M: Post-radiation pleomorphic malignant fibrous histiocytoma of the breast. *Acta Cytol* 30:48–50, 1986.

64. Masin M, Masin F: Cytology of angiosarcoma of the breast; a case report. *Acta Cytol* 22:162–164, 1978.

65. McDivitt RW, Holleb AI, Foote FW Jr: Prior breast disease in patients treated for papillary carcinoma. *Arch Pathol* 85:117–124, 1968.

66. McMahon RFT, Ahmed A, Connolly CE: Breast carcinoma with stromal multinucleated giant cells—a light microscopic histochemical and ultrastructural study. *J Pathol* 150:175–179, 1986.

67. McSwain GR, Valicenti JF Jr, O'Brien PH: Cytologic evaluation of breast cysts. *Surg Gynecol Obstet* 146:921–925, 1978.

68. Mertens HH, Langnickel D, Staedtler F: Primary osteogenic sarcoma of the breast. *Acta Cytol* 26:512–516, 1982.

69. Naran S, Simpson J, Gupta RK: Cytologic diagnosis of papillary carcinoma of the breast in needle aspirates. *Diagn Cytopathol* 4:33–37, 1988.

70. Nguyen G-K, Neifer R: Aspiration biopsy cytology of secretory carcinoma of the breast. *Diagn Cytopathol* 3:234–237, 1987.

71. Norris HJ, Taylor HB: Relationship of histologic features to behavior of cystosarcoma phyllodes; analysis of 94 cases. *Cancer* 20:2090–2099, 1967.

72. Oberman HA: metaplastic carcinoma of the breast; a clinicopathologic study of 29 patients. *Am J Surg Pathol* 11:918–929, 1987.

73. Oertel YC: *Fine Needle Aspiration of the Breast.* Stoneham, Mass, Butterworth, 1987.

74. Ordóñez NG, Manning JT Jr, Raymond AK: Argentaffin endocrine carcinoma (carcinoid) of the pancreas with concomitant breast metastasis; an immunohistochemical and electron microscopic study. *Hum Pathol* 16:746–751, 1985.

75. Orell SR, Sterrett GF, Walters MN-I, Whitaker D: *Manual and Atlas of Fine Needle Aspiration Cytology.* New York, Churchill Livingstone, 1986.

76. Papanicolaou GN, Holmquist DG, Bader GM, Falk EA: Exfoliative cytology of the human mammary gland and its value in the diagnosis of cancer and other diseases of the breast. *Cancer* 11:377–409, 1958.

77. Pearse AGE: Carcinoid of the breast—fact or figment. *Am J Surg Pathol* 1:303–304, 1977.

78. Peters GN, Wolff M: Adenoid cystic carcinoma of the breast; report of 11 new cases: Review of the literature and discussion of biological behavior. *Cancer* 52:680–686, 1982.

79. Pettinato G, de Chiara A, Insabato L, De Renzo A: Fine needle aspiration biopsy of a granulocytic sarcoma (chloroma) of the breast. *Acta Cytol* 32:67–73, 1988.

80. Pietruszka M, Barnes L: Cystosarcoma phyllodes; a clinicopathologic analysis of 42 cases. *Cancer* 41:1974–1983, 1978.

81. Rao BR, Meyer JS, Fry CG: Most cystosarcoma phyllodes and fibroadenomas have progesterone receptor but lack estrogen receptor. *Cancer* 47:2016–2021, 1981.

82. Ravinsky E, Cavers DJ: Cytology of argyrophilic carcinoma of the breast. *Acta Cytol* 29:1–6, 1985.

83. Ro JY, Silva EG, Gallagher HS: Adenoid cystic carcinoma of the breast. *Hum Pathol* 18:1276–1281, 1987.

84. Rupp M, Hafiz MA, Khalluf E, Sutula M: Fine needle aspiration in stromal sarcoma of the breast; light and electron microscopic findings with histologic correlation. *Acta Cytol* 32:72–74, 1988.

85. Sachdeva R, Kline TS: Aspiration biopsy cytology and special stains. *Acta Cytol* 25:678–683, 1981.

86. Salyer WR, Salyer DC: Metastases of prostatic carcinoma to the breast. *J Urol* 109:671–675, 1973.

87. Sandison AT: Metastatic tumours in the breast. *Br J Surg* 47:54–58, 1959.

88. Schurch W, Lamoureux E, Lefebvre R, Fauteux J-P: Solitary breast metastasis: First manifestation of an occult carcinoid of the ileum. *Virchows Arch* 386:117–124, 1980.

89. Schwartz JG, Clark EGI: Fine-needle aspiration biopsy of mycosis fungoides presenting as an ulcerating breast mass. *Arch Dermatol* 124:409–413, 1988.

90. Silverberg E, Lubera JA: Cancer statistics, 1988. *CA* 38:5–22, 1988.

91. Silverman JF, Feldman PS, Covell JL, Frable WJ: Fine needle aspiration cytology of neoplasms metastatic to the breast. *Acta Cytol* 31:291–300, 1987.

92. Silverman JF, Geisinger KR, Frable WJ: Fine-needle aspiration cytology of mesenchymal tumors of the breast. *Diagn Cytopathol* 4:50–58, 1988.

93. Simi U, Moretti D, Iacconi P, et al: Fine needle aspiration cytopathology of phyllodes tumor; differential diagnosis with fibroadenoma. *Acta Cytol* 32:63–66, 1988.

94. Skoog L: Aspiration cytology of a male breast carcinoma with argyrophilic cells. *Acta Cytol* 31:379–381, 1987.

95. Spence RA, MacKenzie G, Anderson JR, et al: Long-term survival following cancer of the male breast in Northern Ireland; a report of 81 cases. *Cancer* 55:648–652, 1985.

96. Stawicki ME, Hsiu J-G: Malignant cystosarcoma phyllodes; a case report with cytologic presentation. *Acta Cytol* 23:61–64, 1979.

97. Stewart FW: The diagnosis of tumors by aspiration. *Am J Pathol* 9:801–813, 1933.

98. Sugano I, Nagao K, Kondo Y, Nabeshima S, Murakami S: Cytologic and ultrastructural studies of a rare breast carcinoma with osteoclast-like giant cells. *Cancer* 52:74–78, 1983.

99. Tavassoli FA, Norris HJ: Secretory carcinoma of the breast. *Cancer* 45:2404–2413, 1980.

100. Taxy JB, Tischler AS, Insalaco SJ, Battifora H: "Carcinoid" tumor of the breast, a variant of conventional breast cancer? Hum Pathol 12:170–179, 1981.

101. Torres V, Ferrer R: Cytology of fine needle aspiration biopsy of primary breast rhabdomyosarcoma in an adolescent girl. *Acta Cytol* 29:430–434, 1985.

102. Volpe R, Carbone A, Nicolò G, Santi L: Cytology of a breast carcinoma with osteoclast-like giant cells. *Acta Cytol* 27:184–187, 1983.

103. Ward RM, Evans HL: Cystosarcoma phyllodes; a clinico-pathologic study of 26 cases. *Cancer* 58:2282–2289, 1986.

104. Wilson SL, Ehrmann RL: The cytologic diagnosis of breast aspirations. *Acta Cytol* 22:470–475, 1978.

105. Yazdi HM: Cytopathology of endometrial adenocarcinoma metastases to the breast examined by fine-needle aspiration. *Am J Clin Pathol* 78:559–563, 1982.

106. Zajdela A, Durand JC, Veith F: Aspect cytologique de quelques variétés particulières d'épithéliomas mammaires. *Bull Cancer* 62:227–240, 1975.

107. Zajdela A, Ghossein NA, Pilleron JP, Ennuyer A: The value of aspiration cytology in the diagnosis of breast cancer; experience at the Fondation Curie. *Cancer* 35:499–506, 1975.

108. Zaloudek C, Oertel YC, Orenstein JM: Adenoid cystic carcinoma of the breast. *Am J Clin Pathol* 81:297–307, 1984.

8

The Clinician's View

THE SURGEON AND NAB

Part 1: Joel Lundy, M.D.

Introduction

In Nassau County, New York, the incidence of breast cancer is over 118.3/100,000 females.[23] This ranks among the highest in the United States. Age-adjusted mortality rates for white females are 36.3/100,000 for Nassau County and 22.5 for the United States as a whole.[22] Therefore, it is essential that all new diagnostic and therapeutic approaches be utilized in women in this geographic area. The following illustrates an approach utilized to obtain data rapidly on a problem case.

A 91-year-old woman with mild congestive heart failure was seen in the office for assessment of a rapidly growing breast tumor. On physical examination there was an 8 × 10-cm firm mass, extending from the areolar border almost to the lateral sternal border and fixed to the skin, with neither axillary nor supraclavicular lymphadenopathy. NAB was performed for (1) diagnosis, (2) immunocytochemistry using monoclonal antibody B72.3, and (3) hormone receptors utilizing monoclonal antibodies to the estrogen and progesterone receptors. Within 6 hours, all this information was available.

A surgeon sees a select group of patients with breast disease. All are symptomatic, with the exception of those who are referred for abnormal mammographic findings alone. From a practical standpoint, the key decision is whether or not an excisional biopsy is required. Many surgeons work with three pieces of clinical information to come to this decision: the history, the physical examination, and the mammogram. There is a fourth procedure that can be extremely valuable, is cost effective, has high sensitivity and specificity, and is done rapidly in the office: ABC.[12,28,32] To utilize this technique, several prerequisites must be met: (1) an understanding of its indications and limitations; (2) familiarity with the technique to ensure adequate diagnostic material; (3) a team relationship with a well-trained cytopathologist; and (4) integration of the new information obtained by ABC with the entire clinical picture. It is dangerous to look at any diagnostic test in isolation.

175

Physiologic Nodularity

A common problem is the woman in her reproductive years referred for either cyclic or persistent lumpiness or nodularity in one or both breasts.[15] The primary care physician may find it difficult to perform an examination, and the mammogram generally shows only dense breasts. If examination discloses neither a dominant nodule nor discrete thickening, the patient is reassured. Additionally, it is helpful to aspirate some of the fibronodular areas or "pseudolump."[27] The benign ABC further confirms the clinical impression that no open biopsy is required and alleviates the patient's anxiety.

The Cystic Mass

In the premenopausal patient, the first question can be, "Is the mass cystic or solid?" If I suspect that the mass is cystic, I will aspirate it. Unless the fluid is bloody, a residual mass remains, or the cyst rapidly recurs after initial aspiration, I do not send the fluid for microscopic examination. In three large series of cytologic evaluations of cyst fluid involving over 1,700 cases, a 1 to 2 percent incidence of carcinoma was reported.[2,11,30] The majority of these cancers were associated with bloody aspirates and/or a residual mass. Although a bright red aspirate may be a traumatic tap, a persistent mass that does not resolve over a period of 3 to 4 weeks of observation should have excisional biopsy even though it may be a hematoma. In general, if a cyst recurs after two aspirations, it should be excised, regardless of the cytologic findings. On rare occasions, a cyst with clear fluid can be malignant.[11]

The Solid Mass in the Premenopausal Patient

Most solid lesions in premenopausal patients are benign. Since surgeons see referred patients, almost all patients with a solid, palpable mass will already have had a mammogram. I do not like to aspirate masses prior to mammography because a traumatic aspirate with a secondary hematoma can create a confusing mammographic picture. If the ABC confirms the benign nature of the lesion, how should this information be utilized? If all four pieces of diagnostic information suggest that the lesion is benign, there is a greater than 98 percent chance that it is benign.[7,14] On the other hand, even excisional biopsy is associated with at least a 1 percent false-negative rate.[26] Although a breast biopsy is a minor surgical procedure, the woman may experience much psychologic trauma until she is sure that the lump is benign. The ABC indicates that the patient can be scheduled for out-patient surgery under local anesthesia because of the slim likelihood of carcinoma.

If the aspirate is suspicious or positive for carcinoma, the approach for biopsy is that of possible segmental mastectomy compatible with breast conservation.[5] If the patient is hospitalized, a frozen section may be indicated, and the specimen should be oriented with sutures and margins inked.

The Solid Mass or Discrete Thickening in the Postmenopausal Patient

In these patients, I utilize NAB to add to the preoperative diagnostic information rather than to indicate whether excisional biopsy should be performed. This is the cancer age group, and the conservative approach is excisional biopsy. If the ABC findings are compatible with a benign diagnosis, and the physical examination and mammogram are not suspicious, I give this reassuring information to the patient and schedule out-patient biopsy under local anesthesia. If the physical examination and mammogram are equivocal and the ABC is suspicious, I tend to expedite the biopsy and approach the lesion as if it were malignant. If all preoperative information suggests carcinoma, I indicate this to the patient and discuss the possible therapeutic options.

The Vague Thickening in the Postmenopausal Patient

Occasionally, a "soft" finding such as an ill-defined thickening in the absence of any mammographic abnormality indicates the need for reexamination in 4 to 6 weeks to evaluate the questionable finding. I have changed my approach in these cases by performing NAB on the initial visit. It provides confirmatory information that the patient will not require immediate excisional biopsy. If I am still in doubt at the follow-up visit, I recommend excisional biopsy.

The Clinically Obvious Cancer and ABC

What is the value of NAB when the physical examination and the mammogram are compatible with carcinoma? It has several advantages even if your institution requires frozen section diagnosis before definitive therapy can be undertaken. A prospective study indicates that a delay between open biopsy and modified radical mastectomy (two-stage procedures) is associated with a greater than twofold increase in wound infections.[1] When a patient has a tumor that is not amenable to breast conservation, the diagnosis can be established and definitive one-stage therapy can be planned through discussion with the patient. Not only does NAB give a rapid diagnosis, but it may help to reduce the incidence of postmastectomy wound infection. Tumors that are potentially amenable to breast conservation can also benefit from ABC diagnosis. The situation can be discussed with the patient in definitive terms, and a preoperative workup can be completed based upon this information. If your institution permits definitive therapy based on positive ABC findings, this is also an obvious advantage.[29]

Mammographic Abnormalities and ABC

Biopsies of occult mammographic lesions result in a malignant diagnosis only 10 to 15 percent of the time in most institutions.[21] Can the number of these biopsies be reduced, establishing a significant cost saving, and still not jeopardize the patient? A stereotactic mammographic apparatus permits a needle to be placed within 0.1 cm of the mammographic finding in over 90 percent of the cases in skilled hands.[4,6] Initial studies performed with this apparatus suggest that excisional biopsies could be reduced by at least 50 percent. This approach holds great promise for ABC in better defining indeterminate mammographic findings (see Chapter 10).

Phenotypic Markers and ABC

Investigational studies have been undertaken to determine if NAB can be utilized in immunoperoxidase assays with monoclonal antibodies to give additional diagnostic and prognostic information.

Can a monoclonal antibody function as a diagnostic adjunct for the cytopathologist? We employed monoclonal antibody B72.3 (MAb B72.3) in immunoperoxidase assays done on Papanicolaou-stained slide specimens from palpable breast masses. MAb B72.3 was obtained by standard hybridoma technology, using a membrane-enriched fraction of a breast cancer metastasis in the liver.[24] Our initial studies indicated a sensitivity and specificity of reactivity of 96 percent.[17-19] It can serve as an adjunct in the diagnosis by ABC of the infiltrating lobular cancers and fibroadenomas with cellular atypism. A pitfall is the occasional cytoplasmic staining of apocrine cells, which can mimic the staining pattern seen in malignant cells (see Plate 2.1). In a prospective study of ABC specimens interpreted by us as suspicious, MAb B72.3 was applied directly to the aspirate. The findings suggest that strong reactivity to this antibody, used in conjunction with the clinical and mammographic findings, can alter the surgical approach to a patient with breast disease[13] (see Plate 2).

Several studies have assessed the value of immunocytochemical localization of estrogen receptors[10,16,20] (see Chapter 11 and Plate 1.5–8). MAb H222 Sp, developed against the MCF-7 human breast cancer cell line, is utilized in these protocols.[9] This methodology has inherent advantages over the biochemical determination of estrogen receptors. Large tissue samples are not required, and the sample consists of pure tumor cells rather than a homogenate that may contain connective tissue and benign epithelium. It is less time-consuming, requires no costly equipment, and appears to correlate well with the biochemical results. With the recent development of a monoclonal antibody to the progesterone receptor[9] this methodology may ultimately replace the biochemical assay.

Conclusion

NAB should be utilized in conjunction with the history, physical examination, and mammography in the diagnosis of breast disease. The diagnostic team consisting of the surgeon, mammographer, and cytopathologist must communicate with each other well to realize fully the advantage of employing these modalities prior to excisional biopsy. The future is particularly exciting, as ABC probably will be utilized to diagnose mammographic lesions and, in conjunction with monoclonal antibodies, will help to define phenotypic markers useful as diagnostic and prognostic tools.

Part 2: Robert D. Smink, M.D.

Indications

The most important dictum in the diagnosis of breast disease is that a *dominant mass must be resolved.* Simplistically stated, masses are either cystic or solid. NAB makes this distinction immediately. *If the mass is cystic and decompresses completely,* no further treatment is necessary. The fluid is then sent for cytologic evaluation, although the cost effectiveness of this procedure is questionable. Most cysts with associated malignant tumor contain bloody fluid or regress incompletely following aspiration, leaving a small palpable mass (see the section on "Cystic Carcinoma" in Chapter 7). Thus, the value of cytology in this setting is nil from a financial standpoint. However, the psychologic value of telling the patient that her fluid will be studied and, subsequently, that the cells are benign is inestimable. Most importantly for diagnosis, the patient should return for clinical reevaluation in 2 weeks. If the cyst has not recurred, tumor in the cyst wall can be ruled out.[3]

For solid or incompletely aspirated masses, NAB is performed. The cytopathologist then renders a diagnosis of malignant, suspicious, benign, or unsatisfactory. Depending on the clinical judgment, those masses labeled unsatisfactory probably should be retested at least once for a more definitive diagnosis. Management of patients based on the other reports is detailed in a later section.

Patients frequently present with a mass, as well as a variable degree of nodularity within the breast parenchyma. An experienced breast clinician will not interpret this mass as dominant. When coupled with cyclic mastodynia, such findings are most compatible with fibrocystic change. Symmetrical, bilateral nodularity in the upper outer quadrants in a woman in the latter half of her childbearing years makes this diagnosis more compelling. This complex of symptoms, however, is extremely variable, and clinical judgment must be applied. Excessive open biopsies are unwarranted, yet failure to diagnose a cancer is unconscionable. NAB, then, is a perfect compromise, combining high diagnostic accuracy with low cost, virtually no morbidity, minimal time investment, and no distortion of the breast for future evaluation. But a word of caution is needed: Clinical judgment must apply, since NAB is only as good as the representation of the cytologic sample and the expertise of the cytopathologist.

Patients occasionally present with a complaint of localized or generalized breast pain. Assuming a normal physical examination with no associated mass, mammography should be performed if the patient is over 35 years old. If the mammogram is negative, the patient should be reassured and an explanation of the causes and treatment of mastodynia outlined. Again, however, NAB provides untold reassurance to the patient in this setting and should be considered as part of the workup.

Other less frequent indications for ABC include nipple discharge and various inflammatory changes. The nipple secretion can be smeared directly onto the slide and the aspiration performed from the retroareolar area if no palpable mass is present. Inflammatory changes include skin edema, erythema, sudden localized or generalized swelling, induration, and peau d'orange. NAB is helpful in these instances, but clinical judgment must again be applied in interpreting the cytologic results and planning further studies or treatment (see the section on "Inflammatory Carcinoma" in Chapter 7).

Mammographic Indications

With widespread screening mammography, patients often present in the surgeon's office with abnormal mammograms and no palpable mass. These abnormal radiologic findings include (1) glandular asymmetry, (2) a definitive nodule, (3) diffuse parenchymal calcifications, and (4) isolated areas of microcalcification. Some lesions, such as diffuse glandular asymmetry and calcifications, may be amenable to the scouting NAB (see the section on "Biopsy Procedure" in Chapter 2). Many, however, are small or deep, making them inaccessible to random aspiration biopsy, and other approaches are indicated (see Chapter 10).

Mammography with glandular asymmetry is often difficult to evaluate and can be a "soft" sign of malignancy. Occasionally, there may be asymmetric thickening which corresponds to the mammographic findings but does not qualify as a dominant mass. We often employ scouting NAB in the area of mammographic concern. If no suspicious cytologic findings are obtained, further support is offered for continued observation. With a high level of suspicion, open biopsy should be performed despite negative cytology.

For benign-appearing nodular densities, ultrasound with NAB can be very helpful in further defining these lesions as either solid or cystic. For cystic lesions, the aspirated fluid is sent for cytologic evaluation. For solid lesions, appropriate follow-up treatment is guided by the results. Because of their great frequency, some practicality must be utilized in evaluating these lesions. The risk of malignancy in smooth-walled mammographic lesions under 1 cm in diameter is very low; thus, these lesions can be safely followed with subsequent imaging. Larger lesions which are ultrasonically cystic can also be observed. In these settings, clinical judgment obviously must be applied and is dependent upon the patient's age, hormonal status, and history of prior similar lesions, as well as the presence of multiple lesions.

Mammographic calcifications are a frequent cause of surgical referral. In situations where the calcifications are diffuse throughout the entire breast or a portion of the gland, scouting NAB can be applied to several areas. A similar approach is used with patients who present with a more discrete area of microcalcifications (see Fig. 6.3). When a diagnosis of malignancy is obtained, therapy can be planned without further biopsy. When the cytology is benign, however, the need for excisional biopsy must be determined by the level of concern generated by the type of calcification. The potential yield of such aspirations may be improved in the future, using mammographic localization techniques to ensure placement of the aspirating needle into the area of microcalcifications. Although somewhat more time-consuming, this approach could conceivably eliminate numerous open biopsies by yielding a greater percentage of definitive results (see Chapter 10).

Applications to Diagnosis

The ultimate diagnostic study, of course, is tissue obtained by open surgical biopsy. NAB provides an extremely accurate and useful form of diagnosis with minimal time, money, and discomfort. Obviously, as with other diagnostic techniques, the accuracy of ABC is directly proportional to:

1. The experience and skill of the individual obtaining the specimen.
2. Proper preparation of the cytologic material by the technologist.
3. The knowledge and interpretative skill of the cytopathologist.

In our recent series based on palpable masses, the sensitivity was 94 percent; and the predictive value of a positive report is 100 percent.[29] By contrast with other diagnostic maneuvers, this level of sensitivity is extremely impressive. The accuracy of physical diagnosis of breast masses by experienced clinicians probably approaches 95 percent, while that of mammography is about 85 percent. Ideally, excisional biopsy is 100 percent accurate. These other techniques are well standardized, however, with excellent clinicians, radiographers, and tissue pathologists in virtually all medical centers. The sensitivity of ABC is less consistent from center to center, but as education and experience expand, a similar standard level of diagnostic accuracy can be anticipated.

A dominant mass with benign ABC requires excisional biopsy for resolution. Benign cytology, although highly predictive, does not absolutely rule out cancer in a dominant mass. The major pitfalls are obtaining representative cytologic samples and the experience of the interpreter. In centers skilled in ABC, the latter pitfall becomes negligible and sampling error determines its sensitivity.

Uses in Patient Counseling

The NAB is extremely helpful in expediting diagnosis and reducing the patient's anxiety. All women presenting with breast complaints are apprehensive. We consider breast masses or mammographic abnormalities a psychologic emergency and arrange office consultation within 1 or 2 days. When indicated, NAB is done at the time of this first consultation. If appropriate, a cytologic diagnosis can be rendered rapidly and the patient informed of the results during this initial visit. Much rapport is gained by this approach. Benign diagnoses given over the telephone are readily accepted and appropriate. However, transmittal of the diagnosis of cancer in this indirect fashion is impersonal and potentially psychosis-inducing. The sensitive physician will take all measures to avoid such situations.

The approach outlined above requires cooperation among the clinician, cytotechnologist, and cytopathologist. Institutions have varying abilities to implement a convenient, expedient, and accurate system. If the clinician is geographically available to the laboratory, the cytotechnologist can come to the physician's office, prepare the material, and return immediately to the laboratory to stain and screen the slides. A cytopathologist then reviews the slide and calls the clinician with a verbal diagnosis. The entire process may take as little as 15 minutes and rarely longer than half an hour. Again, we cannot overemphasize the need for full cooperation and trust between the involved clinical and laboratory personnel.

A common situation concerns the patient who presents with a dominant mass which clinically suggests malignant tumor. The mammogram may be positive but could be nondiagnostic. The NAB is performed, and from the ABC the diagnosis of carcinoma is made. In our experience, no additional tissue sampling is necessary. We caution, however, that clinical judgment must apply. If the surgeon questions the diagnosis on clinical grounds or has less than full confidence in the cytopathologist, an open biopsy *must* precede a definitive operation. Nonetheless, we are frequently comfortable in recommending and performing definitive treatment based on ABC, and proceed immediately with counseling the patient regarding therapeutic options.

Suspicious cytology mandates an open biopsy. In our experience, over 50 percent of these patients will prove to have carcinoma. Clinical impressions can help guide the approach. Either a one-stage or a two-stage biopsy procedure is appropriate. We prefer to perform a one-stage procedure under general anesthesia for patients with malignant disease and to perform open biopsy under local anesthesia for those with benign disease. We thus attempt to individualize our approach based on the clinical impressions. Patient sensitivities and biases must also be considered. Again, ABC is helpful in counseling the patient regarding management, even though the diagnosis is not yet definitive.

When the NAB of a dominant mass reveals benign cells, we reassure the patient that this test is highly predictive. We further explain the need for biopsy and absolute tissue diagnosis. We also warn the patient of the small yet real risk that carcinoma may be ultimately diagnosed. Biopsy is then planned, usually under local anesthesia in an ambulatory setting. Most patients are thus spared the anxiety of the lengthy discussion of major breast surgery.

Management of benign disease is also simplified by ABC. The approach to simple cysts has been discussed. If cytology suggests fibroadenoma, we counsel the patient accordingly and recommend excision. We believe that all dominant masses should be removed. For surgeons advocating observation of these lesions, ABC lends additional support to the safety of this approach. Most importantly, the patient can be immediately reassured of her benign condition, and major anxiety is relieved. When the clinical impression of fibroadenoma is followed by a suspicious or even positive cytologic interpretation, we recommend open biopsy under local anesthesia before planning further treatment. This situation, in our experience, is exceedingly rare.

When fibrocystic change is suspected clinically with compatible mammographic findings, NAB is again performed. If the cytology corroborates the clinical impression, judgment must be based on the relative dominance of the mass. Biopsy is recommended when the area is clearly dominant, but many patients do not require biopsy. Again, patient acceptance or anxiety is considered in making the final decision. The ABC findings thus have a major impact on the clinical management of these patients. Finally, NAB is used in a setting where either the patient or the referring physician needs additional reassurance. The cost, in every sense, is so small that it is clearly justified.

Conclusion

We have found ABC to be essential in the evaluation of breast pathology or symptoms. Clinical judgment must, of course, be applied in all situations to determine its role. Moreover, and most importantly, clinicians must evaluate their own institutional experience with ABC to determine how to apply the cytopathologic diagnoses to patient management. As wider experience and knowledge are developed in this field, we expect ABC to gain an even greater and more generalized application in the management of breast disease.

THE GYNECOLOGIST AND NAB

Kaighn Smith, M.D.

The gynecologist is recognized as the primary physician for women, since many see no other physician. Therefore, the gynecologist's role in early diagnosis of breast cancer, the most common cancer in women, is of primary importance.[31] This importance was recognized by the American Board of Obstetrics and Gynecology in a conference on Breast Disease held in May 1986.[3] Subsequently, the board approved objectives for resident education with respect to breast disease, including the following:

1. Demonstrate inclusion of a properly done breast examination as part of each routine examination.
2. Develop a working relationship with appropriate professional colleagues to provide and coordinate an integrated team approach to the immediate and long-term care of women with breast cancer.
3. Provide counseling and emotional support to patients with breast disease and to affected members of the family.
4. Know the indications, usefulness, and implications of methods for breast biopsy.
5. Know and be able to display an appropriate algorithm of management for a patient who appears with an undiagnosed breast mass.
6. Satisfactorily perform aspiration of a breast cyst.
7. Satisfactorily perform fine needle aspiration (cytology) or core needle biopsy (histopathology) of suspicious breast lesions.
8. Demonstrate an appropriate method to identify the presence of a breast abscess and to establish surgical drainage.
9. Physicians should not practice therapy on the breast without the ability to demonstrate the behavioral, cognitive, and technical skills listed above.

Note that the technical aspect of these objectives requires the obstetric/gynecology resident graduates to perform NAB satisfactorily on any palpable breast lesion. The content of these objectives makes official the role of gynecologists in an area which has been controversial.

Breast lesions have been the province of the general surgeon simply because until mammography and NAB became widely available, the scalpel was the only useful tool to initiate definitive diagnosis of breast cancer. Yet, the gynecologist, with the patient herself, has been the first line of defense in the initial detection of breast cancer. The time has come when gynecologists must practice all diagnostic methods, including NAB.

It is difficult for the gynecologist to keep as high an index of suspicion as the general surgeon, since most breast examinations are for routine annual checkups. Remember, the general surgeon examines the patient only after a breast problem has been found or when there is close follow-up of previously treated breast disease. Often the gynecologist sees the overanxious patient with fibrocystic disease who needs reassurance. Unfortunately, this reassurance too often is given to the patient with early breast carcinoma. The many lawsuits demonstrate the gynecologist's low index of suspicion, the tendency to provide assurance, and the lack of immediate ability to perform a simple needle biopsy. The recent emphasis on education in breast disease for the obstetric/gynecology resident will help us to assume greater responsibility.

There are a number of reasons that the gynecologist must be involved in the accurate diagnosis of breast lesions, using NAB. An important factor is the rapidity with which a diagnosis is made. At our institution, a patient has the diagnosis of a breast mass within 24 hours from the gynecologist. Often the patient has found a breast lump by self-examination. Her immediate reaction is to call her gynecologist.

Her surprise and disappointment are well founded if she learns that the gynecologist does not aspirate breast cysts or do needle biopsies and finds that she must go to a surgeon. The same dismay occurs when the mass is found on routine examination in the office. How easy it is to have the biopsy needle immediately available in order to settle the issue quickly rather than to have her spend anxious hours or days prior to an appointment with the general surgeon.

In the office, the procedure is very simple (see Chapter 2). A brief discussion with the patient, usually while still examining the breasts, informs her that the diagnosis can be determined immediately. Generally, the patient is told that if fluid can be removed, the lesion is benign and the mass will disappear. A question regarding any allergy to the local anesthetic is the only precaution. There are no known contra-indications.

The cyst and the solid lesion can always be distinguished by NAB. The delight and relief of the gynecologist, nurse, and patient when a lesion solid to palpation yields clear yellow fluid and then disappears is one of the joys of our practice. The disappointment in finding abundant tissue to place on the slide after a "gritty" feeling with the needle probe is difficult to hide but must be accomplished until the final diagnosis of malignant tumor is made. "Rushing" the specimen for a definitive diagnosis at least avoids prolonged anxiety.

When fluid is found, it is always sent for cytologic examination, although it is rare to have clear, straw-colored fluid contain malignant cells, and many centers discard such fluid. When no fluid is encountered, at least two needle passes are made. If material appears scant or consists of only fat, three or four samples are taken through the same skin wheal, using the same needle and syringe.

In 1987, at Lankenau Hospital, 21 percent of breast cyst aspirations and 15 percent of solid mass aspirations were done by gynecologists. Of the 142 solid lesions aspirated by gynecologists, 19 percent were reported as unsatisfactory. Further experience and training in the nuances of the technique of NAB and full communication between the cytopathologist and gynecologist should improve this early result.

The team approach to medical problems has never been more important than in the early diagnosis of breast carcinoma.[25] The members of the team in this instance are the patient, the gynecologist, the cytopathologist, the radiologist, and the surgeon. The gynecologist must refer to the surgeon for biopsy as necessary, even in the face of negative ABC findings.

Since women depend on their gynecologist for so much of their care, it has become important for the specialty to broaden its parameters. All aspects of diagnosis of breast disease must be addressed. The performance of NAB by the gynecologist fits perfectly into the specialty.

THE INTERNIST-ONCOLOGIST AND NAB

Christopher P. Holroyde, M.D.

To the hematologist-oncologist accustomed to performing bone marrow aspiration and biopsy, the ease, simplicity, and low cost of NAB should not be surprising.

What is surprising, perhaps, is the fact that only relatively few internists avail themselves of this useful diagnostic technique. In part, this may reflect the general reluctance of internists to encroach upon an area which formally has been the prerogative of surgeons. In part also, it may reflect the lack of suitably trained cytopathologists and a general lack of awareness concerning the ease and speed with which NAB may be performed and a diagnosis rendered.

For an oncologist with a substantial patient population being either treated or followed for breast cancer, the opportunity to utilize NAB as an important diagnostic tool is relatively frequent. Patients who have previously undergone mastectomy, with or without reconstruction, or patients who have undergone an alternative procedure such as lumpectomy with axillary node dissection or radiation therapy are routinely followed by an oncologist when judged to be at risk for the development of locally recurrent or metastatic disease. Many of these patients are either receiving adjuvant therapy or have done so in the recent past. Aside from periodic evaluations to exclude the presence of distant disease, an essential component of the physical examination is the inspection of the chest wall and lymph node drainage areas. Suspicious lesions involving the surgical scar or an adjacent area of the anterior chest wall readily lend themselves to NAB. It should be noted that difficulties encountered in examination of the anterior chest wall are compounded by the presence of surgical prostheses, which represent a particular challenge to the evaluating physician, both clinically and radiographically. The irradiated breast may also undergo progressive retraction and fibrosis, especially in patients with large, fatty breasts. In determining the nature of such contracted and/or nodular tissue, NAB may be particularly helpful and may avoid the need for surgical biopsy, which leads to further scarring. In addition, clinically suspect lymphadenopathy can be readily evaluated by this technique with a high degree of accuracy and with minimal risk (see Chapter 9). It must always be recognized, however, that false negatives can occur, and the potential need for surgical biopsy in situations that are cytologically or clinically suspicious must always be considered.

Because a woman who has diagnosed breast cancer is at risk for developing primary disease in the contralateral breast, annual mammography, clinical examination, and interval self-examination are routine. Palpable, suspicious lesions in the contralateral breast can readily be evaluated by NAB. Because of the simplicity of the technique, the procedure has a high rate of patient acceptability in the follow-up of lesions which are clinically worrisome. With deep-seated lesions or lesions that are too small for easy access, NAB can be performed under mammographic guidance with a higher degree of accuracy (see Chapter 10).

In evaluating possible distant sites of metastases, NAB is particularly useful in the diagnosis of nodular or cystic cutaneous or subcutaneous lesions. Occasionally, surprising findings result, such as soft-tissue sarcoma or metastases from other primary sites. While NAB can be performed on intraabdominal and thoracic masses, these procedures are best performed by the radiologist or surgeon with access to appropriate radiographic guidance.

In conclusion, NAB is a readily available, simple, and inexpensive diagnostic procedure, the skills for which can quickly be mastered by the general internist. As the technique becomes widely accepted and generally available, it should, and no doubt will, be increasingly utilized by hematologist-oncologists and general internists in office practice.

REFERENCES

1. Beatty JD, Robinson GV, Zaia JA, et al: A prospective analysis of nosocomial wound infection after mastectomy. *Arch Surg* 118:1421–1424, 1983.

2. Bell DA, Hajdu SI, Urban JA, et al: Role of aspiration cytology in the diagnosis and management of mammary lesions in office practice. *Cancer* 51:1182–1189, 1985.

3. Conference Proceedings, the American Board of Obstetrics and Gynecology: Conference on breast disease, May 13, 1986. Chicago, 1987.

4. Dowlatshahi K, Jokich PM, Bibbo M, et al: Cytologic diagnosis of occult breast lesions using stereotaxic needle aspiration. *Arch Surg* 122:1343–1346, 1987.

5. Fisher B: Reappraisal of breast biopsy prompted by use of lumpectomy-surgical strategy. *JAMA* 253:3585–3588, 1985.

6. Gent HS, Sprenger E, Dowlatshahi K: Stereotaxic needle localization and cytologic diagnosis of occult breast lesions. *Ann Surg* 204:580–584, 1986.

7. Goodson WH III, Mailman R, Miller TR: Three year follow-up of benign fine-needle aspiration biopsies of the breast. *Am J Surg* 154:58–61, 1987.

8. Greene GL, Fitch FW, Jensen EV: Monoclonal antibodies to estrophilin: Probes for the studies of estrogen receptors. *Proc Natl Acad Sci* 77:157–161, 1980.

9. Greene GL, Harris K, Bova R, et al: Purification of T47D human progresterone receptor and immunochemical characterization with monoclonal antibodies. *Mol Endocrn* 2:714–726, 1988.

10. Keshgegian AA, Inverso K, Kline TS: Determination of estrogen receptor by monoclonal antireceptor antibody in aspiration biopsy cytology from breast carcinoma. *Am J Clin Pathol* 89:24–29, 1988.

11. Kline TS, Joshi LP, Neal HS: Fine needle aspiration of the breast. Diagnosis and pitfalls: a review of 3545 cases. *Cancer* 44:286–292, 1979.

12. Kline TS, Kannan V, Kline IK: Appraisal and cytomorphologic analysis of common carcinomas of the breast. *Diagn Cytopathol* 1:188–193, 1985.

13. Kline TS, Lundy J, Lozowski M: Monoclonal antibody B72.3: An adjunct for evaluation of "suspicious" aspiration biopsy cytology from the breast. *Cancer* in press.

14. Kreuzer G, Boquoi E: Aspiration biopsy cytology, mammography and clinical exploration: A modern setup in diagnosis of tumors of the breast. *Acta Cytol* 20:319–323, 1976.

15. Love SM, Gelman RS, Silen WS: Fibrocystic "disease" of the breast: A non-disease. *N Engl J Med* 307:1010–1014, 1982.

16. Lozowski M, Mishriki Y, Lundy J, et al: Estrogen receptor determination in fine needle aspirates of the breast. *Acta Cytol* 31:557–562, 1987.

17. Lundy J, Kline TS, Lozowski M, et al: Immunoperoxidase studies by monoclonal antibody B72.3 applied to breast aspirates; diagnostic considerations. *Diagn Cytopathol* 2:95–98, 1988.

18. Lundy J, Lozowski M, Mishriki Y: Immunocytochemistry applied to a spectrum of benign and malignant breast aspirates: Strengths and pitfalls. *Br Cancer Res Treat* in press.

19. Lundy J, Lozowski M, Mishriki Y: Monoclonal antibody B72.3 as a diagnostic adjunct in fine needle aspirates of breast masses. *Ann Surg* 203:399–402, 1986.

20. McClelland RA, Berger U, Miller LS, Powlee TJ, Coombes, RC: Immunocytochemical assay for estrogen receptor in patients with breast cancer: Relationship to a biochemical assay and to outcome of therapy. *J Clin Oncol* 4:1171–1176, 1986.

21. Moskowitz M: Minimal breast cancer and redux. *Radiol Clin North Am* 21:93–113, 1983.

22. Nassau County Department of Health.

23. New York State Department of Health, 1982 statistics.

24. Nuti M, Teramoto YA, Mariani-Constantini R, et al: A monoclonal antibody (B72.3) defines patterns of distribution of a novel tumor-associated antigen in human mammary carcinoma cell populations. *Int J Cancer* 29:539–545, 1982.

25. Nyirjesy I, Billingsley FS: Detection of breast carcinoma in a gynecologic practice. *Obstet Gynecol* 64:747–751, 1984.

26. Patchefsky AS, Potok J, Hoch WS, Libshitz HI: Increased detection of occult breast carcinoma after more thorough histologic examination of breast biopsies. *Am J Clin Pathol* 60:799–804, 1973.

27. Patey DH: Two common non-malignant conditions of the breast. *Br Med J* 1:96–99, 1949.

28. Shabot MM, Goldberg IM, Schick P, et al: Aspiration cytology is superior to tru-cut needle biopsy in establishing the diagnosis of clinically suspicious breast cancer. *Ann Surg* 196:122–126, 1982.

29. Sheikh FA, Tinkoff GH, Kline TS, Neal HS: Final diagnosis by fine-needle aspiration biopsy for definitive operation in breast cancer. *Am J Surg* 154:470–475, 1987.

30. Strawbridge HTG, Bassett AA, Foldes I: Role of cytology in management of lesions of the breast. *Surg Gynecol Obstet* 152:1–7, 1981.

31. Wertheimer MD, Castanza ME, Dodson TF, et al: Increasing the effort toward breast cancer detection. *JAMA* 255:1311–1315, 1986.

32. Zajdela A, Ghossein NS, Pilleron JP, Ennuyer A: The value of aspiration cytology in the diagnosis of breast cancer: Experiences at the Fondation Curie. *Cancer* 35:499–506, 1975.

COLOR PLATES

Plate I.1. Mucinous carcinoma. Note pathognomonic cell balls within mucin. Papanicolaou preparation (×125).

Plate I.2. Mucinous carcinoma. Note diffusely scattered tumor cells within mucin. Papanicolaou preparation (×125).

Plate I.3. Metaplastic carcinoma, pseudosarcomatous type. Note spindle cell with red cytoplasm indicating keratin positivity. Immunoperoxidase and hematoxylin preparation for keratin (×500).

Plate I.4. Prostatic carcinoma metastasis to breast. Note acinus with red cytoplasmic granules indicating PAP positivity. Immunoperoxidase and hematoxylin preparation for prostatic acid phosphatase (×500).

Plate I.5. Breast carcinoma, ABC. Estrogen receptor immunocytochemical assay (ER-ICA). Note brown nuclear positivity. Immunoperoxidase and hematoxylin preparation (×500).

Plate I.6. Breast carcinoma, ABC. Progesterone receptor immunocytochemical assay (PR-ICA). Note blue nuclear negativity. Immunoperoxidase and hematoxylin preparation (×500).

Plate I.7. Breast carcinoma, ABC. Progesterone receptor immunocytochemical assay (PR-ICA). Note brown nuclear positivity. Immunoperoxidase and hematoxylin preparation (×500).

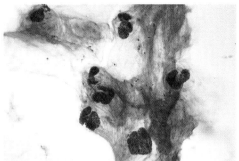

Plate I.1.

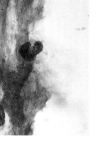

Plate I.2.

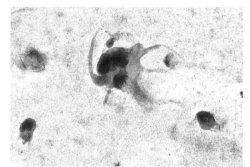

Plate I.3.

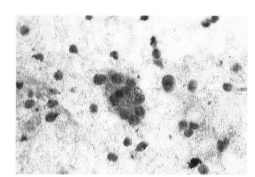

Plate I.4.

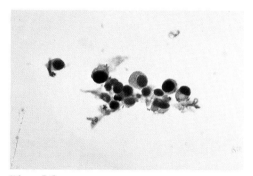

Plate I.5.

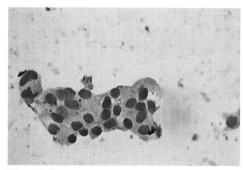

Plate I.6.

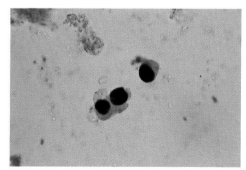

Plate I.7.

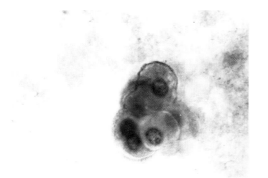

Plate II.1.

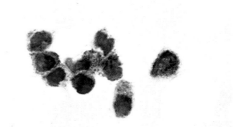

Plate II.2.

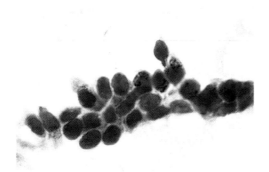

Plate II.3.

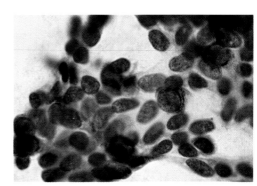

Plate II.4.

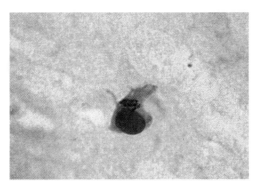

Plate II.5.

Plate II Monoclonal antibody B72.3 (MAb B72.3), ABC Avidin biotin immunoperoxidase technique. Note brown cytoplasmic granules indicating positivity (×1250).

Plate II.1. Apocrine metaplasia. Note intense stain localization on cytoplasmic membrane plus intracytoplasmic staining.

Plate II.2. Infiltrating lobular carcinoma.

Plate II.3. Atypical ductal hyperplasia.

Plate II.4. Lobular carcinoma in-situ.

Plate II.5. Intraductal carcinoma.

9

Post-Tumor Therapy and ABC

INTRODUCTION

Suspected recurrence or metastases in patients treated by mastectomy, lumpectomy, chemotherapy, or radiation should be sampled by NAB as the first procedure. Advantages include the following:

1. It is a rapid, easy, sensitive office biopsy.
2. It distinguishes cancerous nodules of the breast from scar tissue, inflammatory lesions, benign tumors, and secondary neoplasms.
3. A metastasis diagnosed by ABC can be a tumor marker for therapeutic evaluation.

Diagnosis may be more accurate by NAB than by core biopsy. In a comparative study of 51 patients who developed soft-tissue lesions following carcinoma therapy, the false-negative rate of ABC was 13 percent, compared to 44 percent with the histologic section. The ABC findings probably would have been even more reliable had the lesion been sampled by multiple needle passes rather than by a single pass.[13]

LOCALIZED RECURRENT DISEASE

Newly formed lesions at the surgical margins of resection demand investigation. After mastectomy, about 20 percent of patients develop local tumors.[12] Following lumpectomy, 10 percent of 1,108 patients had local recurrence, often adjacent to the original carcinoma.[4] Early diagnosis of these new growths is critical because of the relatively long-term survival; in one series, 45 percent of patients were tumor free 5 years after excision of the isolated nodule.[12]

ABC

Distinction of recurrent disease from foreign body reactions, scar tissue, and inflammatory masses usually can be made by ABC with ease.[10] In irradiated patients,

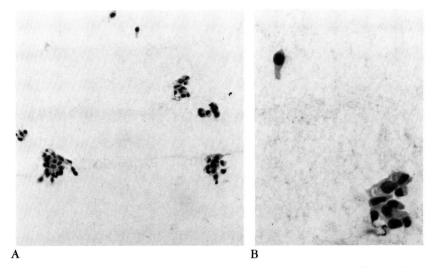

A   B

Fig. 9.1. Mastectomy site, recurrent ductal carcinoma, ABC. **A.** Note the characteristic cell-rich, monomorphic specimen. Papanicolaou preparation (×125). **B.** Higher power. Note the nuclear membrane irregularity and anisonucleosis. Papanicolaou preparation (×300).

however, diagnosis may be difficult (see the section on "Radiation" in this chapter). In most cases, the positive ABC from recurrent tumor reveals all the criteria of malignancy. The cell-rich specimen is monomorphic and dyshesive. The cells show nuclear membrane irregularity, anisonucleosis, and macronucleoli (Fig. 9-1). The pattern and individual cells generally resemble the primary tumor with which they should be compared (see the pertinent descriptions in Chapters 6 and 7).

Scar tissue is the most frequently encountered benign nodule at the resection site. The needle penetrates the lesion with difficulty, and the cell-poor specimen reveals sparse mesenchymal tissue fragments and isolated or cohesive spindle cells with bland nuclei. The ABC may be termed "unsatisfactory" without the team approach.

Nodules formed by inflammatory and foreign body reactions produce a cell-rich, polymorphic ABC with many inflammatory cells, blood, and debris. Fibroblasts, histiocytes, and benign multinucleated giant cells may be present (see Fig. 9.4 and the section on "Interpretative Traps" in Chapter 5).

METASTASES

Metastases may occur early or late in the disease. In Saphir and Parker's autopsy study,[15] they developed up to 33 years after the original diagnosis, and a few were from occult tumors. Lung and lymph nodes, notably axillary and mediastinal, were involved in 65 percent of the cases, bones in 37 percent (generally the spinal column or pelvis), liver in 56 percent, adrenals in 44 percent, spleen in 23 percent, and ovaries in 16 percent of the cases. In a similar report, Warren and Whitham[19] described metastases in almost every bodily site.

Occult ipsilateral mammary carcinomas may be uncovered by investigation of axillary nodes, as occurred in 72 percent of 43 patients with axillary lymphadenopa-

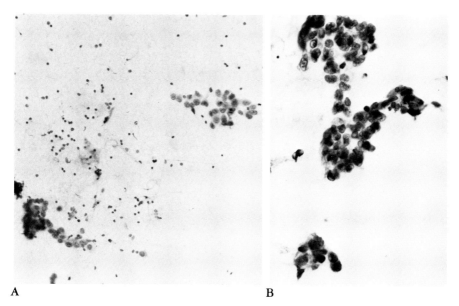

A   B

Fig. 9.2. Occult ductal carcinoma metastatic to the axillary lymph node, ABC. **A.** Note the "alien" cells. Papanicolaou preparation (× 125). **B.** Note the dyshesive aggregates of moderate-sized cells. Papanicolaou preparation (× 300).

thy.[7] The metastases, however, may arise from other tumors. Of 12,302 patients with breast carcinoma, 738 had metastases from a wide variety of nonmammary neoplasms, with many from the uterus and ovary.[16]

Not all suspicious distant masses are malignant. Benign ones include hyperplastic lymph nodes, inflammatory lesions, and benign soft-tissue and skin appendage tumors.

ABC

Metastatic carcinoma is diagnosed chiefly by the presence of cells alien to the site of needle penetration.[9] Therefore, from the application of NAB to the lymph nodes, retrieval of nonlymphoid or "alien cells," aptly named by Söderström[18] usually signifies metastatic tumor.

The majority of the aspirates are cell rich. The ABC may be monomorphic, but when the tumor incompletely replaces the node, alien cells are intermingled with lymphoid cells. They appear in dyshesive clusters or singly, depending upon the histology of the breast carcinoma (Fig. 9.2). Generally, the tumor cells are similar to those from the primary lesions, although they may be more anaplastic. Large, pleomorphic, apocrine-like cells have been described in axillary node metastases from occult breast tumors.[7]

Chemotherapeutic agents may alter both malignant and benign cells. Koss[5,11] probably was the first to document the findings on exfoliated cells. In our experience, viable malignant cells increase in size, with a corresponding enlargement of the increasingly pleomorphic nuclei (Fig. 9.3). Nonviable cells, while larger, display degenerative changes: loss of cytoplasmic and nuclear detail with smudging and

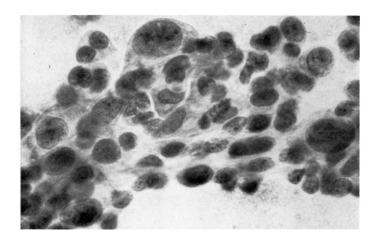

Fig. 9.3. Ductal carcinoma metastasis post chemotherapy, ABC. Note the large tumor cells. Papanicolaou preparation (× 500).

densely hyperchromatic or glassy nuclei. Benign affected cells, sometimes also enlarged and altered in shape, display anisonucleosis and prominent nucleoli; their nuclear/cytoplasmic ratio, however, is considerably smaller than that of malignant cells.

Because of the possibility of a second neoplasm, the tumor cells must be evaluated cautiously. For the cytomorphology of nonmammary tumors, see the section on "Secondary Neoplasms" in Chapter 7). For a complete description of the ABC, contrasting benign and malignant lesions, the reader is referred to the author's *Handbook of Fine Needle Aspiration Biopsy Cytology,* second edition, Chapter 4, "Lymph Nodes and Superficial Masses" (New York, Churchill Livingstone, 1988). Many lesions have special ABC characteristics. Probably the most specific immunocytochemical stain for breast carcinoma is the ER-ICA reaction (see Chapter 11).

RADIATION

Recognition of radiation-induced changes becomes critical because of the increasing use of radiation therapy in conjunction with lumpectomy. Radiation causes cellular alterations which may mimic those of carcinoma and may persist for months or years following treatment. Excisional breast biopsy specimens from 30 patients, 2 months after administration of 6,400 rads, revealed characteristic cellular changes in the terminal ductal-lobular units. The atypical cells of the lobules were distinguished from those of recurrent carcinoma by cellular cohesion and polarity within nondistended lobules.[17]

There are few reports on radiation-induced changes in the ABC. Ruth Graham's classic paper, "Effect of Radiation on Vaginal Cells in Cervical Carcinoma,"[6] remains a valuable resource. The changes in affected exfoliated cells include ballooning with a proportionate increase in nuclear size, cytoplasmic inclusions, and neutrophils. There may be multinucleation, distortion of nuclear membranes, and loss of nuclear detail with hyperchromasia. The seldom-described ABC changes resemble those of exfoliated cells.

Aspirates from irradiated sites often are cell poor. Those from recurrent tumor may display only a few dyshesive malignant cells with ill-defined borders, anisonucleosis, coarse chromatin granules, and some macronucleoli. By contrast, tumor cells inactivated by irradiation or benign cells with radiation-induced changes may be enlarged, with dense, hyperchromatic nuclei and generally no nucleoli.[2,14] The transition between normal and highly atypical cells within a single group or accompanying myoepithelial cells may be signs of benignity. At times, however, distinction between the malignant and benign cells may be impossible. Zajdela et al[20] examined breast aspirates from 202 women 2 years after irradiation. Among 183 patients with active disease, they correctly interpreted 79 percent, classifying 6 percent as suspicious, 2 percent as falsely negative, and 13 percent as unsatisfactory; the ABC from 19 without recurrence was concordant in 80 percent and suspicious in 10 percent; and there were 2 false positives.

INTERPRETATIVE TRAPS

Interpretative traps must be appreciated when these soft-tissue masses are examined by ABC. They include:

1. Geographic miss.
2. Misinterpretation of inflammation, granulation tissue, and fat necrosis.
3. Radiation effect.
4. Heterotopic tissue.
5. Differentiation between carcinoma and benign skin appendage tumors.

Faulty technique causes the majority of false-negative diagnoses. From the NAB of axillary lesions, geographic misses are frequent because of small, mobile lymph nodes buried within fat. In one study,[13] six of seven false-negative diagnoses were made from axillary node metastases. Multiple passes and the team approach to determine needle–node contact lessen the problem.

The ABC findings from inflammatory lesions may mimic those from carcinoma or sarcoma. Cell-rich specimens are common, with isolated, pleomorphic, reactive epithelial cells and histiocytes; nuclei demonstrate anisonucleosis and macronucleoli. Benign multinucleated giant cells generally indicate a benign lesion, but they are also associated with the rare metaplastic carcinoma (see Chapter 7). Correct interpretation is based on the polymorphism, as well as on vesicular, sometimes bean-shaped nuclei with smooth membranes and finely granular chromatin (Fig. 9.4).

Radiation creates many diagnostic problems. A number of cases must be designated as unsatisfactory because of insufficient cells. In one series consisting of superficial soft-tissue nodules, most specimens were placed in this category.[3] Zajdela et al.[20] have concluded that there are no pathognomonic criteria for viability of irradiated tumor cells. Pleomorphism may result in false-positive diagnosis and cell paucity in false-negative interpretation. To prevent these traps, the biopsy procedure must be as vigorous as possible, with multiple passes. When the ABC

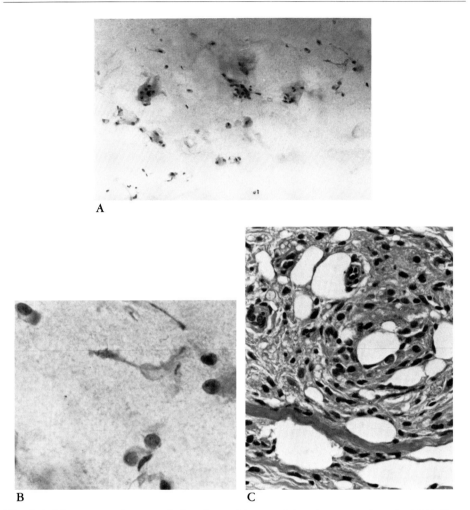

Fig. 9.4. Mastectomy site, granulation tissue: false-suspicious interpretation. **A.** ABC. Note the many loosely connected and isolated cells. Papanicolaou preparation (×125). **B.** ABC, higher power. Note the epithelioid cells with vesicular nuclei. Papanicolaou preparation (×500). **C.** Tissue section. Note the abundant polymorphic cells. Hematoxylin and eosin preparation (×300).

findings are equivocal, the cells must be interpreted as suspicious; thereafter, the NAB can be repeated at 6-week to 6-month intervals until a diagnosis can be made.

Heterotopias may give the erroneous impression of alien cells. Extramammary nodules of breast tissue have been aspirated by us and others.[1,8] We have misinterpreted an endometrioma and an unexpected collection of apocrine cells because of the presence of presumed alien cells.[8] In these cases, the ABC pattern is benign and relatively cell poor. The uniform, bland cells generally are in cohesive bundles, and the cell membranes are distinct. Anticipation of possible heterotopias combined with awareness of the clinical findings is crucial.

Superficial lesions, including cysts and skin appendage tumors, may cause false positives. Knowledge of the ABC characteristics of these benign superficial lesions and the team approach generally prevent mishaps[8] (see the section on "Interpretative Traps" in Chapter 5).

REFERENCES

1. Bhambhani S, Rajwanshi A, Pant L, Das D, Luthra UK: Fine needle aspiration cytology of supernumerary breasts; report of three cases. *Acta Cytol* 31:311–312, 1987.

2. Bondeson L: Aspiration cytology of radiation-induced changes of normal breast epithelium. *Acta Cytol* 31:309–310, 1987.

3. Briffod M, Gentile A, Hébert H: Cytopuncture in the follow-up of breast carcinoma. *Acta Cytol* 26:195–200, 1982.

4. Fisher ER, Sass R, Fisher B, et al: Pathologic findings from the National Surgical Adjuvant Breast Project (Protocol 6); II. relation of local breast recurrence to multicentricity. *Cancer* 57:1717–1724, 1986.

5. Forni AM, Koss LG, Geller W: Cytological study of the effect of cyclophosphamide on the epithelium of the urinary bladder in man. *Cancer* 17:1348–1355, 1964.

6. Graham RM: Effect of radiation on vaginal cells in cervical carcinoma. I. Description of cellular changes. *Surg Gynecol Obstet* 84:153–165, 1947.

7. Haupt HM, Rosen PP, Kinne DW: Breast carcinoma presenting with axillary lymph node metastases; an analysis of specific histopathologic features. *Am J Surg Pathol* 9:165–175, 1985.

8. Kline TS: *Handbook of Fine Needle Aspiration Biopsy Cytology,* ed 2. New York, Churchill Livingstone, 1988.

9. Kline TS, Kannan V, Kline IK: Lymphadenopathy and aspiration biopsy cytology; review of 376 superficial nodes. *Cancer* 54:1076–1081, 1984.

10. Kline TS, Neal, HS, Holroyde CP: Needle aspiration biopsy; diagnosis of subcutaneous nodules and lymph nodes. *JAMA* 235:2848–2850, 1976.

11. Koss LG, Melamed MR, Mayer K: The effect of busulfan on human epithelia. *Am J Clin Pathol* 44:385–397, 1965.

12. Magno L, Bignardi M, Micheletti E, Bardelli D, Plebani F: Analysis of prognostic factors in patients with isolated chest wall recurrence of breast cancer. *Cancer* 60:240–244, 1987.

13. Pedersen L, Guldhammer B, Kamby C, Aasted M, Rose C: Fine needle aspiration and tru-cut biopsy in the diagnosis of soft tissue metastases in breast cancer. *Eur J Cancer Clin Oncol* 22:1045–1052, 1986.

14. Pedio G, Landolt U, Zobeli L: Irradiated benign cells of the breast: A potential diagnostic pitfall in fine needle aspiration cytology. *Acta Cytol* 32:127–128, 1988.

15. Saphir O, Parker ML: Metastasis of primary carcinoma of the breast with special reference to spleen, adrenal glands, and ovaries. *Arch Surg* 42:1003–1018, 1941.

16. Schenker JG, Levinsky R, Ohel G: Multiple primary malignant neoplasms in breast cancer patients in Israel. *Cancer* 54:145–150, 1984.

17. Schnitt SJ, Connolly JL, Harris JR, Cohen RB: Radiation-induced changes in the breast. *Hum Pathol* 15:545–550, 1984.

18. Söderström N: *Fine Needle Aspiration Biopsy.* New York, Grune & Stratton, 1966.

19. Warren S, Whitham EM: Studies on tumor metastasis. 2. The distribution of metastases in cancer of the breast. *Surg Gynecol Obstet* 57:81–85, 1933.

20. Zajdela A, de Maublanc MA, Pilleron JP: La fiabilité de l'examen des tumeurs mammaires par cytoponciton; experience de l'Institut Curie. *Chirurgie* 107:193–198, 1981.

10

Image-Directed NAB for Occult Mammary Lesions

Lydia Pleotis Howell
and Karen K. Lindfors

INTRODUCTION

To screen for breast cancer, the American Cancer Society and the American College of Radiology have recommended mammography annually for women aged 50 or over, every year or two for those between 40 and 49, and as a baseline examination for those between the ages of 35 and 39.[19] As more nonpalpable lesions are discovered, an increasing number of women ultimately may have to undergo surgical biopsy to determine the benign or malignant nature of the mammographically suspicious lesion. Consequently, the utility of NAB for assessment of the nonpalpable lesion is under investigation.

SCREENING MAMMOGRAPHY

Several studies have demonstrated the importance of mammographic screening in the detection of breast cancer. The Health Insurance Plan (HIP) study in the 1960s was the first prospective, randomized, controlled trial to determine if a combination of mammography and physical examination as a screening method could lead to decreased mortality from breast cancer. Results showed that the study group's mortality due to breast cancer was about 30 percent below that of the control group and that this improvement was maintained over 16 years of follow-up.[26-28] Mammography proved to be a valuable screening modality, since the cases that were positive only on mammography had a fatality rate of 14 percent while those that were positive only on physical examination or on both physical and mammographic examination had fatality rates of 32 and 41 percent, respectively.[33]

Randomized, controlled trials to study the effect of mammographic screening alone on breast cancer mortality were also performed in Sweden and Holland. In Sweden, there was a 31 percent reduction in mortality from breast cancer and a 20 percent reduction in the rate of stage II or more advanced breast cancer in the study group. Results from the Dutch study were similar.[34] These studies not only confirmed the results of the HIP study but further emphasized that mortality from breast cancer could be decreased by mammography alone.

The Breast Cancer Detection Demonstration Project (BCDDP), begun in 1973, was intended to make the techniques of early breast cancer detection available to the community. Twenty-nine BCDDP centers were widely distributed throughout the United States, and women were screened annually for a period of 5 years, using the medical history, physical examination, and mammography. These women were then followed for an additional 5 years. In the 50- to 59-year age group, 42.1 percent of breast cancers were detected by mammography alone in the BCDDP, compared to 41.5 percent in the HIP study. However, mammography was positive, either with or without a positive physical examination, in 91.8 percent of the BCDDP breast cancers in this age group versus only 60.0 percent in the HIP study.[2] This difference reflects the improvement in mammographic technology during the interval between the two studies.

Initially in the HIP study, only women over the age of 50 were noted to benefit from screening. A survival advantage, however, became demonstrable after 5 years of follow-up in the 45- to 49-year age group and after 8 years in the 40- to 45-year group. In the BCDDP, mammography alone detected 35.4 percent of the breast cancers and was positive, regardless of the findings of physical examination, in 85.4 percent of the patients in the younger age group, by contrast to only 38.8 percent of the younger patients in the HIP study. At surgery, 89 percent of minimal cancers were demonstrated by mammography in women in the younger age group, 45 percent of which were discovered by this modality alone. Increased mammographic detection in younger women also appeared to improve mortality, since the cumulative 5-year survival rate was significantly lower than the breast cancer mortality in the HIP study.[2] Once again, the improvement in mammographic detection of breast cancer in the BCDDP can be attributed to improvement in mammographic technique.[6] In summary, the HIP, Swedish, Dutch, and BCDDP studies all demonstrate that mammography is an important screening tool in all women over the age of 40 and that it can identify breast cancers at an early stage, thereby decreasing mortality from that disease.

MAMMOGRAPHIC FEATURES OF CARCINOMA

The classic mammographic appearance of breast cancer is that of a dominant mass with ill-defined, spiculated margins (Fig. 10.1). Mammographic visualization of such a mass has a false-positive rate of only 4 percent, but only 14 percent of these cancers will be minimal at the time of diagnosis.[24] Carcinomas may assume more subtle forms: Some will appear as well circumscribed, round, or lobulated masses (Fig. 10.2) or as areas of asymmetry or architectural distortion in comparison to the

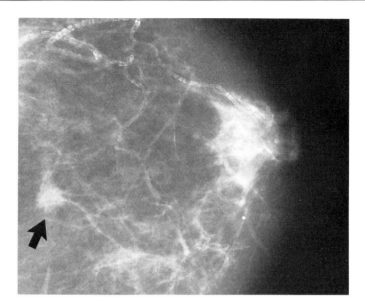

Fig. 10.1. Craniocaudal mammogram demonstrates an 8-mm spiculated mass (arrow) typical of cancer. The pathologic diagnosis was infiltrating ductal carcinoma.

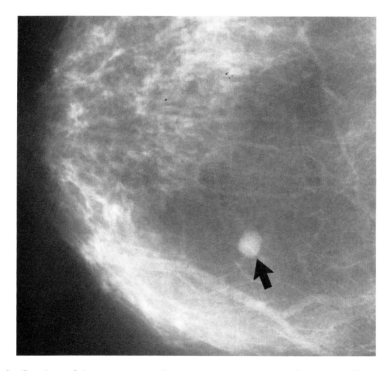

Fig. 10.2. Craniocaudal mammogram demonstrates a 9-mm, well-circumscribed mass (arrow) which was an infiltrating ductal carcinoma.

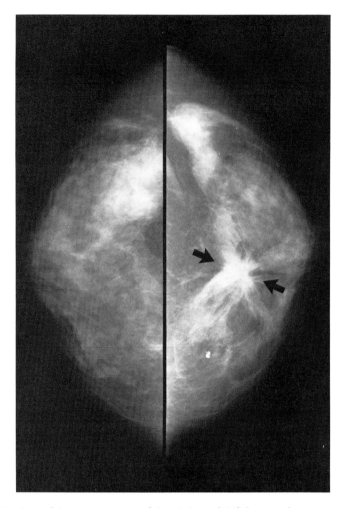

Fig. 10.3. Craniocaudal mammograms of the right and left breasts demonstrate an area of architectural distortion (arrows) centrally in the left breast secondary to infiltrating ductal carcinoma.

opposite breast (Fig. 10.3). A newly developed density in a patient with previous mammograms should also be viewed with suspicion.

The most common mammographic sign of early breast cancer is a cluster of microcalcifications, often without an associated mass. They are small, usually between 100 and 300 μm in size, of varying shapes, and occur in tight groups (Fig. 10.4).

Unfortunately, many benign processes present a mammographic appearance which overlaps that of carcinoma. Therefore, while mammography is a very sensitive examination, it is not very specific for breast cancer. A biopsy of clustered microcalcifications detects 71 percent of minimal cancers but has a false-positive rate of 88 percent.[24] As a consequence, many surgical biopsies are performed on nonpalpable, benign lesions. The true-positive biopsy rate for nonpalpable breast carcinomas ranges between 20 and 30 percent,[10,11] and may be as low as 10 percent in aggressive

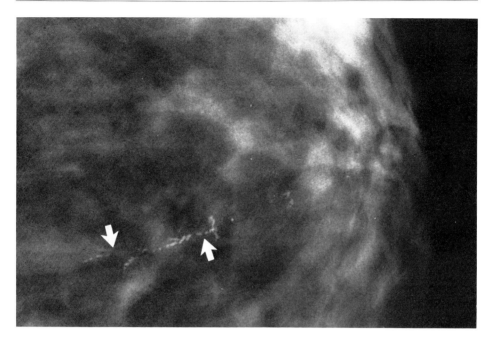

Fig. 10.4. Magnified view of malignant microcalcifications (arrows) (infiltrating ductal carcinoma). Note that there is no associated mass.

programs.[24] Nonetheless, aggressive mammographic screening is still cost effective.[22] An alternative to surgical biopsy, particularly in indefinite lesions, is mammographic follow-up, but many clinicians are reluctant to take this course because of fear of litigation.

NAB

Since NAB of palpable breast masses has been shown to be highly accurate, and more safe and cost effective than surgical biopsy, many investigators have been studying NAB of nonpalpable breast lesions directed by a variety of imaging modalities. The results from these studies are summarized in Table 10.1 and are discussed below.

Stereotaxic Devices

A stereotaxic instrument developed in Sweden allows sampling of nonpalpable breast lesions with a precision of ± 1 mm. The patient lies prone on a tabletop, with her breast protruding through a circular hole. Two plates with a square aperture marked with coordinates compress the breast from below at the desired angle. An x-ray tube on a hinged arm that can be inclined at different angles is attached to a pivot stand that can turn the tube, puncture device, and compression plate in a semicircle. Once adjustments are made so that the lesion is visible within the coordinate system, radiographs are taken at different angles. From the resulting stereoradiographs,

TABLE 10.1. Nonpalpable Lesions and NAB: Statistics from the Literature

Author	Total	Method	% Unsatisfactory	Sensitivity	False Positive	False Negative
Bibbo et al.[3]	114	Stereo.	13.2% (15/114)	93.3% (14/15)	—	—
Fornage et al.[7]	51	U/S	?	100% (12/12)	—	—
Gent et al.[8]	187	Stereo.	11.7% (31/187)	97.5% (39/40)	—	2.5% (1/40)
Kehler and Albrechtsson[12]	182	Mammo.	26.9% (49/182)	100% (41.41)	16.8% (15/92)	0
Lindfors et al.[17]	34	Mammo.	2.9% (1/34)	91.7% (11.12)	—	10% (1/10)
Nördenström and Zajicek[25]	23	Stereo.	—	100% (5/5)	—	—
Svane and Silfversward[30]	120	Stereo.	7.5% (9/120)	85.7% (48/56)	3.6% (2/55)	14.2% (8/56)

coordinates to the center of the lesion are determined. The biopsy is then taken with the puncture device.[4] Use of both the screw needle[21,30] and the simple needle[31,8] has been reported.

Results with this stereotaxic instrument have been very good. Lesions composed of suspicious clusters of microcalcifications and masses of soft tissue density have been sampled by this method. Studies have shown that the amount of cellular material obtained, while usually adequate for diagnosis, has an unsatisfactory rate of 7.5–11.7 percent.[3,8,30]

One series showed a 3.6 percent false-positive rate[30] while all others have shown none. False-negative results ranging from 2.5 to 14.2 percent have been reported.[8,30] Most series indicate a sensitivity ranging from 85.7 to 97.5 percent,[3,8,30] though Nördenström and Zajicek reported 100 percent accuracy in the diagnosis of malignant and benign breast lesions with this device.[25]

A smaller, less expensive stereotaxic system for NAB recently has been developed. The biopsy apparatus consists of cassette and needle holders and a measurement device that calculates the respective coordinates for the lesion and needle holder. This device fits on two currently marketed mammographic units (GE senographe 500T and 600T, Milwaukee, WI) and is reported to allow placement of a biopsy needle within 0.1 cm. The precision of the system was tested on 107 mammographic examinations: A specific diagnosis of a cyst, fibroadenoma, carcinoma, or lymph node was possible in 42 cases, but false-positive and false-negative results were not reported.[5]

Sonography

Sonography has proven to be ineffective as a screening method for breast carcinoma.[15] Breast ultrasound currently is used mainly to differentiate cystic from solid masses (Fig. 10.5). For nonpalpable lesions, the demonstration of a cyst is diagnostic, and further workup is usually unnecessary. If confirmation is desired, ultrasound-guided aspiration of the cyst can be performed.[7,14]

Ultrasound has been used to guide NAB of nonpalpable solid masses. Fornage et al.[7] obtained positive cytology in all 12 of their aspirated breast carcinomas, but there was one false-positive report. Since their series included palpable masses, the number of unsatisfactory specimens from clinically occult lesions is unclear.

Ultrasound offers the advantages of no radiation exposure and equipment which is readily available in most radiology departments. The position of the tip of the biopsy needle relative to the lesion is easy to document with this modality. Recent reports, however, indicate that only 58 to 65 percent of cancers are seen sonographically.[15,29]

Mammography

At the University of California, Davis, we are studying NAB of nonpalpable breast masses directed by mammography.[17] As with ultrasound, the equipment is readily available in most radiology departments. Many radiologists are already familiar with the necessary technique, since it is similar to needle localization of clinically occult lesions for surgical biopsy. NAB requires an alert, cooperative patient who has not been sedated. The point of entry for the biopsy needle is determined by review of craniocaudal and lateral mammograms. Either the craniocaudal, mediolateral, or

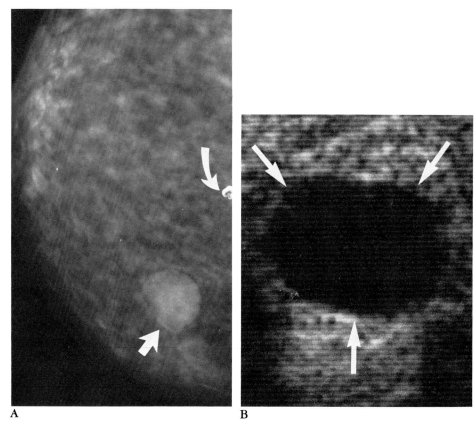

Fig. 10.5. Craniocaudal mammogram (**A**) in an asymptomatic patient demonstrates a 1.5-cm, partially circumscribed mass medially (arrow). Benign calcifications (curved arrow) were also noted. Sonogram (**B**) shows a cyst (arrows).

lateromedial approach may be used. If the x-ray tube will swing 180 degrees, the caudocranial approach can be used, but this is somewhat awkward, and in most cases the next closest skin surface will be used as a point of entry to inferior lesions. The patient's breast should then be placed in the mammography unit in the position that will allow the radiologist access to the skin surface closest to the lesion.

Most currently available dedicated film screen mammographic units are equipped with guidance systems that facilitate accurate positioning of biopsy or localizing needles. The guidance system usually involves the use of a fenestrated compression paddle (Fig. 10.6). The paddle may contain a single large fenestration that is marked along the edges with radiopaque grid lines, or it may have multiple holes, each of which is identified with radiopaque numbers and/or letters. A paddle with a single large fenestration is preferable for NAB, as it allows exact positioning of the needle and rotation of the x-ray tube while the needle protrudes through the fenestration.

The breast is compressed by the fenestrated compression plate, and a film is exposed. The patient must remain in the compressed position while the film is developed. After the film is received, the coordinates of the lesion are plotted and marked on the skin.

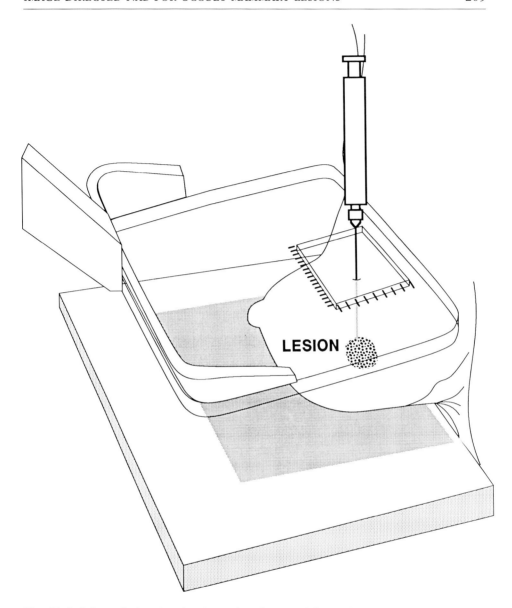

Fig. 10.6. Schematic drawing showing NAB of an occult breast lesion using mammographic guidance. A fenestrated compression plate with grid lines is used to guide the placement of the biopsy needle. The needle is placed through the opening, perpendicular to the patient's skin and parallel to the x-ray beam. The film cassette is located beneath the breast (shaded area).

The skin is cleansed with Betadine solution. Local anesthesia is generally not used. A 22- or 25-gauge needle long enough to reach the lesion is inserted perpendicular to the skin and parallel to the x-ray beam. A film is then taken to ensure proper needle position in this axis. If the lesion can be felt with the tip of the needle during this pass, NAB can then be taken in that area (Fig. 10.7). For experienced personnel, the time for completion of the procedure approximates 20 to 30 minutes.

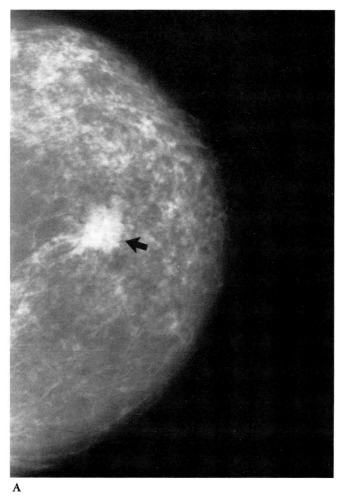

A

Fig. 10.7. Left craniocaudal mammogram (**A**) shows a suspicious lesion (arrow) at 12 o-clock. A coned craniocaudal view (**B**) in preparation for NAB shows the lesion to be within the fenestration at the intersection of lines drawn from "F" and "2.5" on the marked grid. A similar view (**C**) shows a 25-gauge spinal needle which was inserted parallel to the x-ray beam and perpendicular to the patient's skin entering the lesion. The lesion was easily felt with the needle tip. (**D**). ABC, infiltrating ductal carcinoma. Papanicolaou preparation ×500.

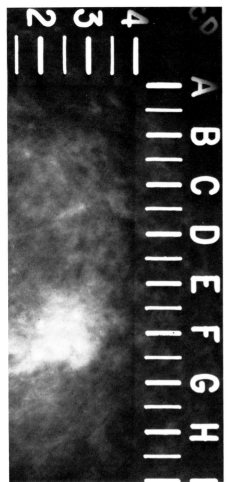

B

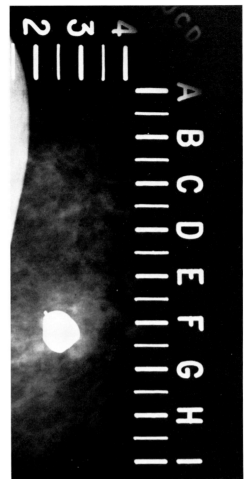

C

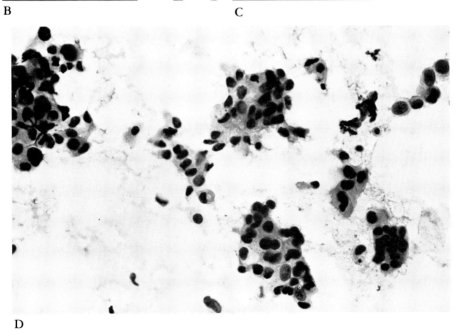

D

207

If the lesion is not palpable with the needle tip, the needle should be advanced to a point beyond the lesion. Then a film should be taken to ascertain that the needle transfixes the lesion. The compression is then carefully released, and the x-ray tube is angled slightly. The fenestrated device is again used for compression, and a film is exposed. The projected total length of the needle is then measured, as is the distance from the lesion to the needle tip. A simple geometric ratio [(true needle length/projected needle length) × projected distance of tip to lesion] can be used to determine the actual distance from the needle tip to the lesion. The needle tip can then be retraced so that it is in the lesion, and an aspiration biopsy can be obtained (Fig. 10.8). We choose only suspicious masses of soft tissue density for aspiration,

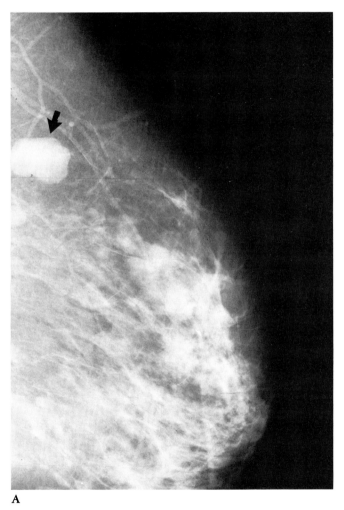

A

Fig. 10.8. Left mediolateral mammogram (**A**) shows a 2.2-cm lobulated mass (arrow) in the upper outer quadrant. This mass had enlarged since the previous mammogram. A coned view (**B**) with the fenestrated compression plate in place shows the needle directed toward the lesion. Since the lesion could not be felt with the needle tip, the patient was placed in a lateral position, and the mammogram (**C**) shows the needle to be within the lesion. (**D**). ABC, fibroadenoma. Papanicolaou preparation, × 300.

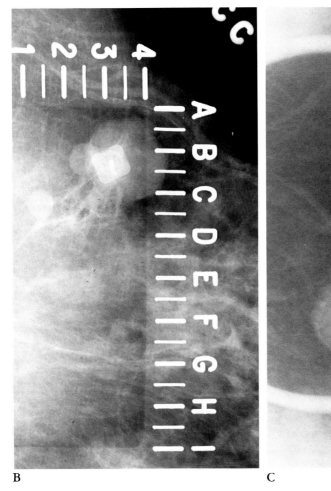

B

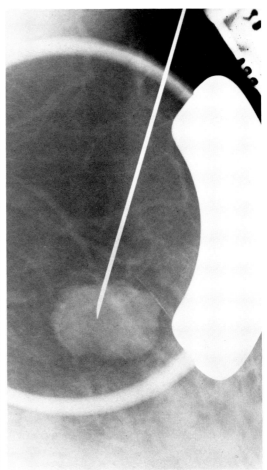

C

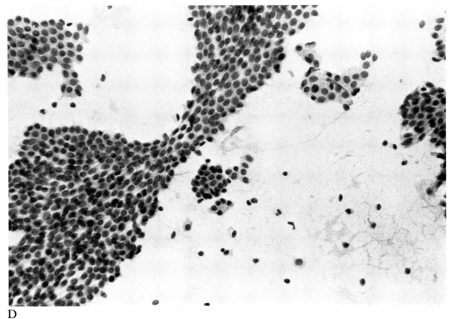

D

209

since these have a higher likelihood of being malignant or of being a lesion with a characteristic cytologic pattern, such as a fibroadenoma. Eleven of 12 carcinomas were correctly identified as suspicious or positive. Sensitivity was 91.7%, in the range of what has been reported for the stereotaxic method.[17] Kehler and Albrechtsson performed 182 NABs using a similar method, and demonstrated a sensitivity of 100 percent.[12] Similar studies have shown a concordance of 94 percent between the ABC and surgical biopsy.[18]

Diagnostic Problems

A problem inherent in NAB of occult lesions, regardless of the modality used, is inability to stabilize the lesion. In both the intramammary lymph nodes and some of the fibroadenomas we sampled, the aspirating needle could be felt to be deflected from the smooth, well-circumscribed, mobile mass (Fig. 10.9). As a consequence, the specimen was actually from the adjacent breast parenchyma. Svane and Silfversward[30] experienced a similar problem with the Swedish device, which disappeared with increased experience. The problem of lesion displacement by the needle may be unique to certain benign masses, since this sensation has not been observed during aspiration of any malignant lesions.[13,30] Perhaps the reactive fibrosis created by the crab-like infiltrating carcinoma sufficiently anchors it for easier penetration by the fine needle.

Unsatisfactory specimens secondary to scant material can be a problem and may be due to characteristics of the lesions themselves. In our study, some fibroadenomas in postmenopausal women yielded only a few benign ductal cells because of dense, hyalinized stroma. Similar cytologic findings were seen in a patient with a scar from a previous breast biopsy. Although carcinoma with a dense scirrhous reaction can also lead to a cell-poor aspirate and can be a potential cause of a false-negative diagnosis, this was not a problem in our single case of infiltrating lobular carcinoma.

The technique required to aspirate nonpalpable masses may also affect the cellularity of the specimen. We observed that the smears are often less cellular than those obtained from palpable masses. While in a large, palpable mass the needle must be directed into multiple areas during aspiration to obtain a representative sample and increase the cellular yield, this is not possible in a tiny, nonpalpable lesion. Decreased cellularity has also been noted in specimens obtained by the Swedish instrument and is attributed to the rigid fixation of the needle necessary for precision.[3]

Role in Clinical Decision Making

How does the clinician use the information obtained from NAB of clinically occult lesions (Fig. 10.10)? When a carcinoma is diagnosed, the clinician can counsel the patient and plan definitive treatment. If a mastectomy is the treatment of choice, the patient can proceed directly to this operation. An intervening excisional biopsy or frozen section has thus been avoided and with it the associated extra cost, risk, and worry to the patient. However, cytologic evaluation of a malignant breast lesion does not yield information regarding the infiltrating nature or extent of the disease. If the choice of a lumpectomy is contingent on this information, needle localization and surgical biopsy may have to be performed. Armed with the cytologic diagnosis,

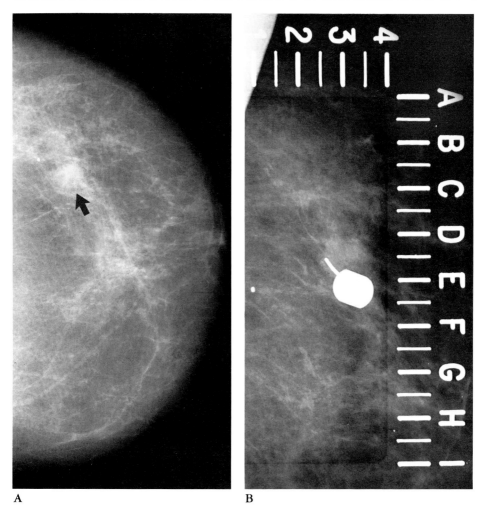

A   **B**

Fig. 10.9. Left mammogram (**A**) showing a suspicious, ill-defined lesion in the upper outer quadrant (arrow). A craniocaudal coned view (**B**) shows the NAB needle sliding off the periphery of the lesion. Despite repeated attempts at NAB, the lesion could not be penetrated. The ABC demonstrated fibroadipose tissue. Surgical excision revealed a fibroadenoma.

however, the surgeon can do an excisional biopsy with adequate margins and an axillary dissection during the same operation, potentially obviating the need for further surgery.

For certain benign lesions, including cysts, fibroadenomas, and lymph nodes, surgical excision need not be performed. The characteristic cytologic pattern can lead to a definite diagnosis of fibroadenoma. Carcinoma associated with fibroadenoma is very rare.[9] When cyst fluid is aspirated, the image-directed NAB is not only diagnostic but also therapeutic. The lesion should be reimaged to ascertain complete collapse (see the section on "Cystic Carcinoma" in Chapter 7). We have correctly interpreted the findings from seven benign cysts and two fibroadenomas.

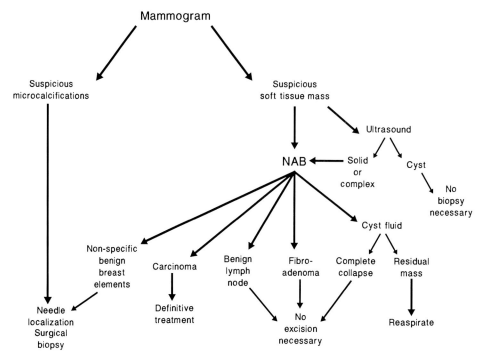

Fig. 10.10. Decision tree summarizing the clinical approach to the evaluation of suspicious occult breast lesions.

The question remains as to how reliable radiologically directed NAB is when only nonspecific benign breast elements are obtained. Svane[31] investigated possible false-negative diagnoses from the stereotaxic technique, potentially the most precise method of localization. In his series, 306 patients with benign cytologic findings were followed mammographically for periods ranging from 4 to 49 months. The lesions in 297 patients either diminished in size or remained unaltered on follow-up mammography, confirming their benign nature. Four of the nine patients, who underwent eventual surgical excision because of radiologic enlargement or other clinical considerations, had a malignant tumor. In Kehler and Albrechtsson's series,[12] 89 cytologically benign lesions were followed by clinical, cytologic, and mammographic reexamination over a 4- to 59-month period, with no carcinoma uncovered.

These findings appear to indicate that NAB of clinically occult breast lesions can give a meaningful benign diagnosis. Confidence in sampling, however, remains a haunting problem. In a palpable lesion, where the aspirator can stabilize the mass manually, and see and feel if the needle penetrates it, both the pathologist and the clinician may judge that a few benign ductal cells and fibroadipose tissue represent a nodule of fibrocystic change. These clinical features, which inspire confidence, are not present when nonpalpable lesions are aspirated.

The team approach is essential for the evaluation of the clinically occult lesion. The cytologic findings must be correlated both with the mammographic appearance of the lesion and with the radiologist's degree of certainty that the biopsy needle tip was in the lesion. Suspicious microcalcifications on mammography pose a particularly difficult problem. Identification of calcifications in the aspirate is the only way the pathologist can confirm that the correct area has been sampled. With uncertainty that the lesion was adequately sampled, the patient should undergo open biopsy. A nonspecific cytologic interpretation from NAB of an occult breast lesion does not eliminate the need for follow-up mammography. Subsequent diagnosis of carcinoma, while rare, does occur. We suggest that if a mammographic lesion carries such a low degree of suspicion that open biopsy would not be recommended, a patient should have the customary follow-up mammogram rather than NAB.

In summary, we believe that NAB of occult breast lesions currently is useful in two situations: One is the definitive diagnosis of a benign lesion with a characteristic cytologic pattern so that the need for surgical biopsy is obviated. The other is a positive diagnosis of carcinoma so that definitive surgery can be carried out without intervening surgical biopsy.

REFERENCES

1. American College of Radiology: Guidelines for mammography. Policy statement. Reston, Va, September 22, 1982.
2. Baker LH: Breast Cancer Detection Demonstration Project: Five-year summary report. *CA* 32:194–225, 1982.
3. Bibbo M, Scheiber M, Cajulis R, et al: Stereotaxic fine needle aspiration cytology of clinically occult malignant and pre-malignant lesions. *Acta Cytol* 32:193–201, 1988.
4. Blomgren J, Jacobson B, Nördenström B: Stereotaxic instrument for needle biopsy of the mamma. *Am J Roentgenol* 129:121–125, 1977.
5. Denarnaud Y, Haehnel P, Isnard A, Chaintreuil J: Stereotactic breast puncture: New step in breast screening. *Diagn Imaging* 189–192, 1987.
6. Eddy D: *The Value of Mammography for Women Under 50.* New York, American Cancer Society, 1986.
7. Fornage BD, Faroux MJ, Simatos A: Breast masses: US-guided fine-needle aspiration biopsy. *Radiology* 162:409–414, 1987.
8. Gent HF, Sprenger E, Dowlatshahi K: Stereotaxic needle localization and cytological diagnosis of occult breast lesions. *Ann Surg* 204:580–584, 1986.
9. Goldman RC, Friedman NB: Carcinoma of the breast arising in fibroadenomas with emphasis on lobular carcinoma: A clinicopathologic study. *Cancer* 23:544–550, 1969.
10. Hall F: Screening mammography—potential problems on the horizon. *N Engl J Med* 314:53–55, 1986.
11. Homer M: Non-palpable breast abnormalities: A realistic view of the accuracy of mammography in detecting malignancies. *Radiology* 153:831–832, 1984.
12. Kehler M, Albrechtsson U: Mammographic fine needle biopsy of non-palpable breast lesions. *Acta Radiol Diagn* 25:273–276, 1984.
13. Kline TS, Joshi LP, Neal HS: Fine needle aspiration of the breast, diagnosis, and pitfalls: A review of 3545 cases. *Cancer* 44:286–292, 1979.
14. Kopans DB, Meyer JE, Lindfors KK, Bucchianeri, SS: Breast sonography to guide cyst aspiration and wire localization of occult solid lesions. *AJR* 143:489–492, 1984.
15. Kopans DB, Meyer JE, Lindfors KK: Whole breast US imaging: Four-year follow-up. *Radiology* 157:505–507, 1985.

16. Kopans, DB, Waitzkin ED, Linetsky L, et al: Localization of lesions identified in only one mammographic view. *AJR* 149:39–41, 1987.

17. Lindfors KK, Howell LP, Russell LA, Hartling R: Unpublished data.

18. Mahsood S, Frykberg ER, McLellan G, et al: Potential value of mammographically guided fine-needle aspiration biopsy in assessment of non-palpable lesions. *Am J Clin Pathol* 89:437, 1988.

19. *Mammography: Two Statements of the American Cancer Society.* New York, American Cancer Society, 1983.

20. Meyer JE, Kopans DB, Stomper PC, Lindfors KK: Occult breast abnormalities: Percutaneous preoperative needle localization. *Radiology* 150:335–337, 1984.

21. Moskowitz M, Fox SH: Cost analysis of aggressive breast cancer screening. *Radiology* 130:253–256, 1979.

22. Moskowitz M: Screening is not diagnosis. *Radiology* 133:265–268, 1979.

23. Moskowitz M, Gartside PJ: Evidence of breast cancer mortality reduction: Aggressive screening in women under age 50. *AJR* 138:911–916, 1982.

24. Moskowitz M: Minimal breast cancer and redux. *Radiol Clin North Am* 21:93–113, 1983.

25. Nördenström B, Zajicek J: Stereotaxic needle biopsy and preoperative indication of non-palpable mammary lesions. *Acta Cytol* 21:350–351, 1977.

26. Shapiro S: Evidence on screening for breast cancer from a randomized trial. *Cancer* 39:2772–2782, 1977.

27. Shapiro S, Venet W, Strax P, Venet L, Roeser R: Ten-to-fourteen year effect of screening on breast cancer mortality. *JNCI* 69:349–355, 1982.

28. Shapiro S, Venet W, Strax P, Venet L, Roeser R: Screening, follow-up, and analysis in the Health Insurance Plan Study: A randomized trial with breast cancer screening. *Natl Cancer Inst Monogr* 67:65–74, 1985.

29. Sickles EA, Filly RA, Callen PW: Breast cancer detection with sonography and mammography: Comparison using state of the art equipment. *AJR* 140:843–845, 1983.

30. Svane G, Silfversward C: Stereotaxic needle biopsy of nonpalpable breast lesions: Cytologic and histopathologic findings. *Acta Radiol Diagn* 24:283–288, 1983.

31. Svane G: Stereotaxic needle biopsy of non-palpable breast lesions. A clinical and radiologic follow-up. *Acta Radiol Diagn* 24:385–390, 1983.

32. Tabar L, Gad A, Holmberg HL, et al: Reduction in mortality from breast cancer after mass screening with mammography. *Lancet* 1:829–832, 1985.

33. Thomas LB, Ackerman LV, McDivitt RW, et al: Report of the NCI Ad Hoc Pathology Working Group to review the gross and microscopic findings of breast cancer cases in the HIP study. *JNCI* 59:495–541, 1977.

34. Verbeek ALM: *Population Screening for Breast Cancer in Nijmegen: An Evaluation of the Period 1975–1982.* Publication of the Department of Social Medicine, Katholieke Universiteit, Nijmegen, the Netherlands, 1985.

11

Hormone Receptors and Other Tumor Markers

Albert A. Keshgegian

INTRODUCTION

The detection of marker molecules in tumors has been an important advance in recent years. The ability to determine changes in a cell by immunochemical, biochemical, or cytochemical techniques adds a dimension of information not available by standard histopathology or cytopathology. In breast pathology, this type of information could be used potentially in several ways:[61] (1) to classify a poorly differentiated tumor (e.g., carcinoma vs. lymphoma); (2) to identify the primary site of a tumor; (3) to provide information on the prognosis or optimal therapy; and (4) to determine whether a tumor is benign or malignant.

Many marker molecules have been studied in breast carcinoma by a number of techniques. Although most approaches have utilized biochemical or immunochemical methods in analyzing tissue, such methods have also been applied, or potentially could be applied, to ABC specimens. The most extensively studied and most widely used markers are hormone receptors. In this chapter, the usefulness of hormone receptor measurements will be discussed in detail, followed by an overview of other tumor markers in breast cancer.

HORMONE RECEPTORS

Although receptors for a variety of hormones have been studied in breast cancer, the determination of estrogen receptor (ER) and progesterone receptor (PR) has been found to provide the most significant clinical information on the choice of the therapeutic approach, as well as information on the prognosis. Furthermore, the demonstration of ER in a metastatic tumor can be helpful in establishing the breast as the primary site.

The existence of a hormonal relationship in breast cancer has been known for a long time. In the nineteenth century, Beatson[9] showed that breast cancer can regress after oophorectomy. In this century, it has been found empirically that removal of hormones by oophorectomy, adrenalectomy, or hypophysectomy, or addition of hormones in pharmacologic doses, will cause remission of metastatic breast cancer in some patients.

These findings have been at least partially explained by studies on steroid hormone metabolism.[57,141] In contrast to peptide hormones, which have a receptor on the cell membrane and activate a second messenger in the cytoplasm, steroid hormones enter cells. In the cells of sensitive organs, there are protein receptors for the steroid hormone. These protein receptors are characterized by very high binding affinity for the correct steroid and by high specificity—other steroid hormones bind to the receptor with much less affinity than the proper hormone. Thus, the receptor is capable of accumulating the specific hormone within cells of sensitive organs even though the outside concentration is low. When the steroid hormone has combined with the protein receptor, the receptor in the complex becomes activated and acquires the ability to bind to the chromatin-DNA material at specific sites. The mechanism of specific binding is only poorly understood but may involve nonhistone proteins that are part of the chromatin complex. Specific new messenger RNA species are synthesized and, from them, specific new proteins. The new protein species are characteristic of the hormone and the target organ.

The receptor traditionally has been measured by homogenizing a tissue specimen, obtaining a cytosol supernatant by ultracentrifugation, and determining the amount of binding in the supernatant to radioactively labeled hormone.[141] For the measurement of ER, labeled estradiol is used. In the most commonly used method, increasing concentrations of estradiol are added to aliquots of the cytosol, followed by adsorption of nonbound estradiol onto dextran-coated charcoal and determination of the nonadsorbed (and thus receptor-bound) radioactivity. The data are analyzed by Scatchard plot for the number of receptors and the characteristic dissociation constant. In another method, the hormone–receptor complex is centrifuged in a sucrose density gradient, and the radioactivity that migrates at the characteristic size range of the receptor (and is thus bound to the receptor protein) is determined. Values are expressed as femtomoles (10^{-15} moles) of receptor per milligram of cytosol protein. Values above 3–10 fmol/mg are considered positive for breast tumors.

Since normal breast tissue contains small amounts of ER, breast tumors may also contain the receptor if the capability to synthesize it has not been lost in the course of malignant differentiation. Jensen[55,57] suggested that tumors that are likely to respond to hormonal therapy should contain the receptor protein for estrogen, whereas tumors that do not contain the receptor should be hormone insensitive. This prediction generally has been borne out.[141] Numerous studies have shown that the frequency of response in ER-positive women for ablative therapy or hormonal additive therapy (depending on the menopausal status of the patient) ranges from about 55 to 60 percent. In contrast, the response rate in women whose tumor is estrogen receptor negative is less than 10 percent. The measurement of estrogen receptor thus is a significant tool in predicting which women are likely to respond to hormonal therapy and in identifying women in whom chemotherapy should perhaps be attempted first.

However, the predictive ability of the ER assay is far from perfect. There are a small number of false negatives (women with tumors negative for ER that do respond to hormonal therapy) and a large number of false positives (women with tumors positive for ER that do not respond). There are several possible reasons for these discrepancies. First, there may be inaccuracies in the receptor measurements.[112] The biochemical assays are technically complex and poorly standardized. Variability can occur between laboratories or even in the same laboratory in multiple measurements on the same specimen. Another explanation is tumor heterogeneity.[101] Different portions of a given breast tumor may be heterogeneous in receptor content; in one area, tumor cells may be rich in ER, whereas in other areas of the same tumor, cells may lack appreciable ER content. Thus, a portion of the tumor that is measured for ER may give a different result, and respond differently to hormonal therapy, than another portion of the tumor that is not measured.

A third explanation for the inexact correlation between ER measurements and the response to hormonal therapy is that in the malignant cell there may be some defect in the steps required for estrogen action after hormone binding.[54] Consequently, new protein products are not synthesized, even though ER is present and able to bind estrogen. The measurement of PR, which is a protein synthesized in response to the action of estrogen, was advocated as a means of increasing the predictive ability of ER measurements.[54] Indeed, if a tumor is positive for both ER and PR, the response rate is higher than if it is positive for ER alone.[141] However, even with PR measurements, the response rate is still not close to 100 percent, and some women whose tumors contain ER but lack PR[141] do respond. Therefore, the presence of PR in a tumor adds predictive information, but our ability to predict the probability of a response to hormonal therapy still needs improvement. Also, tumors with higher concentrations of ER are more likely to contain PR and to respond to hormonal therapy than tumors that contain low concentration of ER.[27,52,102] Thus, the quantitative determination of ER may yield information in addition to measurement of both ER and PR.

In addition to providing information on optimal therapy, the presence of hormone receptors in a breast tumor correlates with the prognosis and with other parameters known to affect the prognosis. Well-differentiated tumors or those that occur in older women are more likely to contain hormone receptors[125] and to have a better prognosis[13,55] than poorly differentiated tumors or those in younger women. The presence of hormone receptors also correlates directly with a longer disease-free interval and possibly with longer survival,[12,20,49,69,110] at least in patients who have lymph node metastases.[36]

Hormone receptors also can be used to identify the breast as the primary site of a metastatic adenocarcinoma. Although there are reports of ER-like proteins in many types of tumors,[64] the presence of a high level of ER, along with the appropriate histologic appearance, is evidence of origin from a tissue that is involved in hormone action, e.g., breast, uterus, or ovary.[65]

Biochemical assays for hormone receptors are time-consuming, expensive, and cumbersome, and require substantial amounts of tissue or cells. This has led to attempts at histochemical and immunohistochemical approaches for receptor measurement. These methods all detect the attachment of estrogen-binding proteins in tissue sections to estrogen that is labeled in some way.[26,77,95,109] In the simplest of these approaches, estrogen compounds are labeled directly, e.g., with a fluorescent molecule. Alternatively, labeled anti-estrogen antibodies that putatively bind to the estrogen–protein complex have been utilized. Although proponents of these methods have reported good correlation with results obtained by standard biochemical assay results or with the clinical response, others have failed to find a strong correlation with the biochemical assay.[26,83,105] Histochemical methods also have been criticized for requiring high concentrations of estrogen that would bind not only to high-affinity ER, but also to other estrogen-binding proteins of low affinity (type II sites).[17] Consequently, histochemical methods that rely on detecting bound estrogen must be viewed with skepticism and require extensive further validation.

Recently, a totally different approach for ER measurement has been created with the development of monoclonal antibodies directed against the ER protein itself.[44] With such a monoclonal antibody, immunochemical measurements of ER can be performed on frozen tissue sections or ABC specimens without the need for biochemical binding of estrogen. Numerous studies have shown good correlation between the antibody method and the traditional biochemical assay.[28,50,51,60,66,84–86,104,107,118] There is also preliminary evidence that ER determinations by the monoclonal antibody technique may correlate better with the hormonal response than ER determined by the biochemical assay.[84,107]

In the traditional model of ER action, the receptor resides in the cytoplasm and translocates to the nucleus only after binding estrogen. Unexpectedly, the monoclonal antibody assay has consistently detected ER only in the nucleus[67] rather than in the cytoplasm. This finding has contributed to reexamination of the cytoplasmic model and to the hypothesis that ER is actually a loosely bound nuclear protein that becomes tightly bound to the chromatin material after estrogen binding.[56] Thus, the monoclonal antibody technology may change not only the methods for clinical measurement of ER, but also basic research into the mechanisms of ER action.

HORMONE RECEPTORS IN ABC

Hormone receptor measurements traditionally have been performed on tissue biopsy specimens. Since the diagnosis of breast carcinoma by ABC is reliable, the surgeon can proceed directly to mastectomy without a tissue biopsy.[119] This simplifies the process for the patient but raises the issue of how to obtain material for hormone receptor determinations. Although the mastectomy specimen itself can be used, provided that it is handled expeditiously,[14] it would be advantageous to be able to perform the determinations on the ABC specimen. This would be simpler and quicker, and could provide prognostic information for patient counseling even prior to surgery. It would also be useful in cases of inoperable tumors; for determination of hormone receptors in small metastases; or sequentially to follow the effect of therapy on receptor concentrations.

Early studies by European investigators described biochemical approaches to ABC specimens. Poulsen et al.[111] applied a standard dextran-coated charcoal-binding method. Although they were able to demonstrate ER positivity in some ABC specimens, the sensitivity was much lower than that obtained with tissue. They attributed the low sensitivity in ABC specimens to the low protein concentration in the cytosol extract due to insufficient numbers of cells or to nonrepresentative aspirations.

Silfversward and co-workers[121–123] reported greater success with a method using isoelectric focusing on polyacrylamide gels to identify receptor bound to radioactively labeled estrogen. This more sensitive method showed good correlation of ER values in a cellular aspirate (more than 10^6 cells) with determinations performed on the corresponding tissue. However, a substantial number of aspirates had inadequate material for reliable receptor measurement. The authors recommended the technique primarily for inoperable tumors, which usually yield abundant material on NAB.

Benyahia et al.[10] reported on a dextran-coated charcoal procedure using high-salt extraction of cells. They also found a lower limit of approximately 10^6 cells for reliable ER measurement, an amount that was achieved in 76 percent of their cases. The same group, using similar methodology, also reported reliable measurement of PR in 89 percent of cases.[96] In addition, they measured both ER and PR in the same sample, using a single concentration of radioactively labeled estrogen and a synthetic progesterone analog, with separation by high-pressure liquid chromatography.[90]

Although these studies suggest some success in applying biochemical binding assays to ABC specimens, the methods are technically demanding and tedious, and not applicable for general use. They attempt to obtain maximal information from a small sample, and require approaches such as single-point binding assays that do not provide binding constants and are more subject to variability than multipoint assays performed on tissue. Even with these attempts to increase sensitivity, some ABC specimens still are insufficient for analysis.

Histochemical methods for ER and PR, similar to those in tissue specimens, have also been applied to ABC specimens[25,46,73] and serous effusions.[138] The results show some correlation with results of biochemical binding assays and with longer survival of the patient. However, the use of these techniques on cytologic specimens is subject to the same criticisms as their use on histologic sections.

Methods using antibody against the receptor protein hold the most promise for determination of hormone receptors in ABC specimens. Some investigators have reported on polyclonal anti-ER antibodies that have been developed in their own laboratories.[24,127] However, most investigators have used the monoclonal antibody discussed earlier in this chapter. One group has employed this antibody in an enzyme immunoassay (ER-EIA Estrogen Receptor Enzyme Immunoassay, Abbott Laboratories, North Chicago, IL), using cytosol extracts of cells from ABC specimens, and has concluded that the immunoassay method is more sensitive than biochemical binding assays on ABC specimens;[91] they have not compared the technique with assays on tissue specimens. This approach, even though potentially feasible, still requires homogenization and extraction steps. Accordingly, a more popular approach uses the same monoclonal antibody in an immunocytochemical assay (ER-ICA Estrogen Receptor Immunocytochemical Assay, Abbott Laboratories, North Chicago, IL), which can be performed on ABC specimens ejected onto specially coated glass slides. This technique, similar to other immunocytochemical procedures, is easy to perform and allows assessment of the ER content of individual cells on the glass slides. Specific cells that are malignant by standard ABC criteria can be examined, and the proportion of ER-containing malignant cells can be determined. A disadvantage is that the degree of positivity of an individual cell, reflected by the intensity of staining, is subjective, and the results are at best semiquantitative.

Several groups have used ER-ICA on ABC specimens. Except for one group

TABLE 11.1. Sensitivity and Specificity of ER Determined by ER-ICA on ABC and
Tissue Specimens Compared with Biochemical Assay on Tissue from
the Same Tumor

	ER-ICA: ABC	ER-ICA: Tissue
Sensitivity*	82% (42/51)	88% (43/49)
Specificity†	80% (20/25)	89% (25/28)

*Percentage of cases positive by biochemical assay that are also positive by ER-ICA.

†Percentage of cases negative by biochemical assay that are also negative by ER-ICA.

Source: Keshgegian et al.[63]

which used aspirates taken during clinical evaluations,[23,87] the ABC specimens were
obtained from excised tumors,[37,80,139] tumors immediately prior to surgery,[16,115,116]
or tumors obtained in an unclear manner.[3] These studies have reported 80–100
percent sensitivity and 60–89 percent specificity for ER-ICA on ABC specimens
compared with biochemical assay of tissue[3,37,139] or a lower sensitivity or specificity
for ER-ICA on ABC specimens compared with ER-ICA on tissue specimens.[87,115]

These ABC specimens generally were obtained under artificial circumstances. In
contrast, we have examined the usefulness of ER-ICA performed on ABC specimens taken by surgeons during the initial office diagnostic evaluation of a breast
mass.[63] For this study, surgeons obtained an extra aspiration specimen, in addition to
the two or three for routine examination. Aspirates were brought immediately to
the clinical laboratory, smeared onto glass slides coated with "tissue adhesive" sup-
plied in the ER-ICA kit, briefly fixed, and stored as described by the manufacturer.
Specimens that were positive for carcinoma were stained within 4 weeks by a
peroxidase–anti-peroxidase procedure as described in the ER-ICA kit. Results were
compared with those of biochemical assay of tissue subsequently removed at surgery
and with those of ER-ICA performed on tissue.

Positivity consisted of a brown-colored immunoperoxidase reaction produced in
the nuclei of tumor cells. Positive staining was usually apparent at $100\times$ and readily
verified at $400\times$ (see Plate 1.5). In some specimens, light brown cytoplasmic staining was present, even in negative controls that had been incubated with nonimmune
serum; this was interpreted as nonspecific negative staining. The cellularity of ER-
ICA-stained ABC smears was equal to or somewhat less than that of companion
smears processed routinely with Papanicolaou stain. In a few cases, even though the
number of cells on the Papanicolaou-stained smear was sufficient for cytologic diagnosis of carcinoma, the ER-ICA-stained smear contained inadequate cellularity for
determination of ER content.

The sensitivity and specificity for ER-ICA positivity in ABC specimens compared
to biochemical assay were 82 percent and 80 percent, respectively, whereas for ER-
ICA positivity in tissue the sensitivity and specificity were 88 percent and 89 percent, respectively (Table 11.1). The results show that ER can be determined by ER-
ICA on ABC specimens obtained during initial diagnostic evaluation, with a
sensitivity and specificity approaching those of ER-ICA performed on tissue sections.

The sensitivity of ER-ICA performed on ABC specimens and tissue indicated
occasional false-negative results on both types of specimens compared with the

TABLE 11.2. Scoring System for ER-ICA Positivity

Grade	Positive Cells (%)	Average Nuclear Stain Intensity
0	0–10	Absent
1	10–25	Slight
2	25–50	Distinct
3	50–75	Dark
4	>75	

Note: Score = grade % positive cells + grade intensity.
     (0–7)   (0–4)   (0–3)
Source: Keshgegian et al.[63]

results of biochemical assay. Interestingly, in five cases where there was a discrepancy in results between ER-ICA performed on an ABC specimen and tissue from the same patient, the biochemical assay was invariably positive. This suggests that false-negative ER-ICA results may be caused by degradation of the receptor in material processed for ER-ICA assay even when the recommended procedure is followed.

The specificity data also indicate false-positive ER-ICA results compared with those of the biochemical assay. Results that are positive by ER-ICA but negative by biochemical assay could be due to several causes: (1) heterogeneity of ER in different parts of a tumor, as discussed in the previous section; (2) degradation of receptor in tissue processed for biochemical assay; and (3) measurement of antigenic proteins by ER-ICA that are not extracted for biochemical assay or that cannot bind estrogen. These possibilities require further investigation.

We also attempted to correlate the degree of ER-ICA positivity in ABC specimens with the quantitative biochemical binding value. Although immunoperoxidase values are not quantitative, a semiquantitative estimate can be obtained by combining a grading of the number of positive cells and the intensity of staining. We constructed a simple grading system for the percentage of positive cells and the average intensity of positively stained nuclei. The sum of the two components gives an ER-ICA score ranging from 0 to 7 (Table 11.2). For example, an ABC specimen that contained distinctly brown-colored nuclei (grade 2) in 25–50 percent of tumor cells (grade 2) would have an ER-ICA score of 4. The ER-ICA score correlated roughly with the quantitative biochemical values ($r = 0.45$, $p < 0.001$), although there was much scatter and correlation was insignificant if only the results positive by both assays were considered. A similar approximate correlation has been obtained by other investigators on ABC and tissue specimens, some with more elaborate scoring systems.[37,50,107,139]

ER-ICA positivity also correlates with the histologic grade of the tumor and with the patient's age, factors that correlate with biochemical ER positivity and with the clinical course. ER-ICA positivity, like biochemical ER positivity, is lower in poorly differentiated tumors and in tumors from younger women. Such tumors are also more likely to pursue an aggressive clinical course.

These results establish the feasibility of ER-ICA staining of diagnostic ABC specimens and show correlations with other important parameters in breast carcinoma. However, the most important question is whether ER-ICA measurements predict the eventual hormonal response and the prognosis. There are also the problems of sample procurement (sufficient cellularity, ER lability), lack of quantitation, and measurement of PR by immunocytochemical methodology. Some of these questions are being addressed. There are recent reports of antibodies prepared against PR[51,68,106,108] and of the predictive ability of ER and PR measured by immunocytochemistry on fine-needle aspirates[38] (see Plate 1.6, 1.7). There are also reports on optimizing cell collection in ABC specimens[33] and on computerized image analysis for quantitation of immunocytochemical staining.[4,11] Approaches such as these, as well as the eventual development of antibodies reactive against fixed or partially degraded receptor, may be important developments in making the immunocytochemical measurement of receptors in ABC specimens a clinically valid and reliable technique.

TUMOR CLASSIFICATION

Antigens other than ER have been studied in establishing the epithelial nature of a breast tumor or the breast as the primary site of a metastatic tumor. Most approaches have been immunocytochemical. The principles of using immunochemical procedures to make decisions about breast tumors are similar to those used in other tumors.[61] The antibody should be characterized on known specimens; antibodies from different sources raised against the same putative antigen may stain with different patterns or intensity. One should be certain that the apparent staining of the antigen is actually in malignant cells and not in benign cells, necrotic cells, or macrophages. Staining should be present in known positive controls processed together with the unknown specimen and absent in negative controls, consisting of a second slide of the unknown incubated with nonimmune antiserum. The type of fixation and processing of the specimen can affect substantially the immunochemical results. Most studies of breast tumor antigens have been performed on tissue sections. Cytologic slides, which are fixed and processed differently, may not give the same pattern of reactivity as tissue sections.[18]

One should not rely on the staining results of a single antigen. Instead, one should construct a differential diagnosis and use a panel of antisera, some of which would be expected to be positive in the type of tumor under consideration, and others positive in other types of tumor. For example, in poorly differentiated tumors of the breast, the differential diagnosis may include carcinoma, lymphoma, and melanoma. Positivity for one or more of the generally applicable epithelial markers—epithelial membrane antigen, cytokeratin, or carcinoembryonic antigen (CEA)[61]—is evidence of an epithelial tumor, whereas such tumors should be negative for leukocyte common antigen, a marker for lymphoma,[72] and usually negative for S-100 protein, a marker for melanoma.[98] Conversely, lymphoma or melanoma should contain leukocyte common antigen or S-100 protein, respectively, and should also be negative for epithelial markers. Carcinomas *may* contain S-100 protein,[98] but they should also be positive for one or more epithelial markers, unlike melanoma.[32]

In epithelial tumors, neuron-specific enolase is evidence of neuroendocrine differentiation;[128] however, this antigen can be present in breast carcinomas without other evidence of neuroendocrine features.[99,140] The presence of gross cystic disease fluid protein (GCDFP-15) is a marker for apocrine differentiation.[35,94]

In exfoliative cytologic material, immunochemical staining for epithelial antigens such as CEA,[138] keratin,[113] and epithelial membrane antigen[48] can demonstrate breast cancer cells in serous effusions and increase the diagnostic yield of cytologic examinations.[48] Keratin has also been demonstrated in a few ABC specimens from the breast[29] (see Plate 1.3). In ABC specimens, staining for CEA has been correlated with positivity in tissue sections.[97] In one ABC specimen, positivity for epithelial membrane antigen in a spindle-cell tumor gave support to the diagnosis of carcinoma rather than sarcoma,[40] whereas in another case, osteoclast-like cells in osteoclast-type carcinoma were negative for keratin and CEA and apparently were of nonepithelial origin.[47]

Alpha-lactalbumin, a protein found in milk secretions of breast epithelial cells, has been extensively investigated as a marker for breast origin of a metastatic neoplasm. In immunochemical studies of tissue, approximately 50 to 75 percent of breast tumors have been reported to contain this antigen.[5,21,76,79,136,137] One study, however, failed to detect lactalbumin in any of 44 breast carcinomas, even though some of the tumors were from pregnant or lactating women in whom the benign breast tissue was positive.[6] The reasons for this discrepancy are not clear. False-negative results could be caused by low sensitivity of the antiserum or technique; false-positive results could be due to cross-reaction of some antisera with antigens other than lactalbumin. We have attempted to stain tissue sections for lactalbumin in lactating breasts and breast tumors, with inconsistent results. In one report using ABC specimens, lactalbumin was negative in two breast carcinomas.[132]

In addition to sensitivity in breast carcinomas, there is also the question of specificity. Is staining absent in nonbreast carcinomas? Various adenocarcinomas, predominantly gastrointestinal and lung, have been reported as negative for lactalbumin.[5,21] Lee et al.[76] confirmed this observation but found reactivity with skin appendage and salivary gland tumors and mesotheliomas that apparently was due to antibodies cross-reacting with some material other than lactalbumin. Another study found reactivity in one of four colon carcinomas.[79] Reactivity has also been reported in 19 percent of ovarian epithelial neoplasms.[30]

Thus, although lactalbumin may be useful in demonstrating the breast to be the primary site of a carcinoma, the results are not consistent and the sensitivity and specificity do not approach the high level of markers known to be useful in a comparable organ—prostate acid phosphatase or prostate-specific antigen in prostate carcinoma[62] (see Plate 1.4). The availability of monoclonal antibodies, with reproducible reactivity, may solve some of these problems.

TUMOR PROGNOSIS

The association of ER and prognosis has already been discussed. Although there have been reports of a correlation between other antigens, such as CEA, pregnancy-specific beta$_1$-glycoprotein, and human placental lactogen,[53,92,120] other careful studies have failed to confirm such an association.[8,75] Similarly, other standard antigens, such as lactalbumin, human chorionic gonadotropin, casein, or ABH blood group isoantigens do not correlate with the prognosis.[8,53,74,76,135] There are reports on the correlation of other antigens with the prognosis or the histologic differentiation: pregnancy-associated plasma protein A,[70] transferrin receptor,[142] substances bound by lectins,[39] and milk fat globule membrane-associated antigens recognized by various monoclonal antibodies.[34,45,114] A 52,000-dalton protein, demonstrated on ABC specimens as well as tissue, may correlate with tumor proliferation.[16] An antigen present only on proliferative cells, recognized by monoclonal antibody Ki 67, appears to correlate with the mitotic index and inversely with the ER status.[7,42] These antigens all require more study and confirmation.

Another class of markers that may correlate with tumor prognosis consists of cellular oncogenes, also called "proto-oncogenes," and their protein products.[41] Cellular oncogene products appear to function in normal growth and differentiation. If the oncogene is altered in some way, such as in position, nucleotide sequence, or number of gene copies (amplification), it may be activated inappropriately or excessively; in this situation, rather than promoting normal growth, the functioning protein product appears to contribute to the development of malignant tumors. In human breast cancer, amplification of an oncogene termed HER-2/neu (or c-erb B-2) can be detected by biochemical DNA analysis and correlates with a poor prognosis.[124] Since high levels of the protein product measured immunohistochemically correlate with gene amplification,[134] the potential exists for predicting the prognosis based on the immunohistochemical presence of the oncogene product. A structurally similar and possibly related protein, epidermal growth factor receptor, also correlates with a poor prognosis.[117] The p21 product of the ras oncogene is detectable in both malignant and benign tissues, although the amount generally is higher in malignant tissue.[1,15,19,43,130] Loss of an allele for the ras oncogene in breast carcinoma correlates with tumor aggressiveness.[129] In addition to determining the prognosis, oncogene analysis potentially could be used for tumor detection or classification.[41]

A very different approach used to determine the prognosis is analysis of the DNA content of a tumor. The two DNA-related parameters commonly studied are the proliferative rate of the tumor and the presence of an abnormal (aneuploid) amount of DNA in tumor cells. The proliferative rate has been determined by measuring the incorporation of radioactively labeled thymidine into the DNA of tumor cells; the thymidine-labeling index correlates with the probability of relapse.[89] The DNA content has been measured with dye-binding techniques in ABC, as well as in histologic specimens; the presence of more normal DNA patterns correlates with a better prognosis.[2]

The advent of flow cytometry provides the ability to perform these kinds of studies more quickly and easily. In a flow cytometer, cells in suspension interact individually with a light beam as they flow by rapidly in single file.[22] Many cells can be analyzed rapidly. Light scatter gives information on cell size and other parameters; fluorescence of bound dyes or labeled antibodies can give information on cellular constituents. The instrument can measure readily the DNA content of a cell. It gives the fraction of DNA that it is in the synthetic phase of the cell cycle (S-phase fraction; cell cycle analysis). This measurement correlates with the thymidine-labeling index and the proliferative rate.[89] DNA aneuploidy can be measured much more effectively than with previous methods. Aneuploid breast tumors, as measured by flow cytometry, have a worse prognosis than tumors with a normal (diploid) content of DNA.[31,89] A high proliferative rate and aneuploidy, regardless of the methodology used, also correlate with other poor prognostic factors such as absence of hormone receptors and lack of histologic differentiation.[31,89]

Hormone receptors also potentially could be measured by flow cytometry. Although there are reports on the determination of ER by this technique,[103,133] these studies utilize the controversial labeled-ligand approach discussed above. Whether a technique using labeled monoclonal antibody can be developed remains to be determined.

Flow cytometry is theoretically readily applicable to ABC material,[22] since the cells are already in suspension. Successful application of flow cytometry to demonstrate aneuploidy in ABC specimens of breast carcinoma has in fact been reported[78] (see Chapter 12).

MARKERS FOR MALIGNANT TUMORS

Most tissue-specific antigens cannot be used as evidence of malignant rather than benign proliferation. They are found normally in cells of a particular tissue. Since malignant tumors express some of the same antigens as their normal counterparts, and since well-differentiated tumors are more likely to express these antigens than poorly differentiated ones, the presence of such antigens in a malignant tumor provides evidence only of the tissue of origin or potentially of the clinical course and prognosis. The presence of oncofetal antigens, such as CEA[71] or other antigens newly defined by monoclonal antibodies,[88] may correlate with malignancy; these associations require further study.

The specificity of an interesting monoclonal antibody, termed B72.3, raised against tumor-associated glycoprotein has been investigated. In tissue sections, the antibody reacts strongly with a substantial proportion of breast carcinomas or other carcinomas, but not with normal or lactating breast tissue; it does react weakly with some benign breast lesions.[100,131] This antibody could be utilized as an adjunct to the diagnosis of carcinoma in effusions,[59,93,126] although the more conventional epithelial or oncofetal antigens are also useful for this purpose.[61]

The reactivity of B72.3 antibody has also been studied in ABC specimens. Johnston et al[58] examined formalin-fixed, paraffin-embedded cell blocks of fine-needle aspirates. They found positivity in 81 percent of breast carcinomas but only in 1 of 10 benign breast lesions, restricted to cells from apocrine metaplasia. The results on ABC specimens correlated with staining on tissue subsequently removed surgically. Lundy et al.[82] examined formalin-fixed smears of aspirates performed on surgically excised specimens. They obtained both sensitivity and specificity of 96 percent, with one fibroadenoma showing focal staining; they concluded that B72.3 positivity can increase the sensitivity for the diagnosis of carcinoma. Lundy and co-workers[81] also obtained high accuracy on ABC specimens previously stained by the Papanicolaou technique, with sensitivity of 90 percent for infiltrating lobular carcinoma and specificity of 95 percent (see Plate 2). Although these results are impressive, they should be interpreted with caution. The antibody has been used only by a limited number of investigators and at different dilutions. Furthermore, interpretation is subjective, since "blush"[58] or "1 + "[82] staining was scored as negative. Thus, the reproducibility of these results in other laboratories is not assured.

CONCLUSION

The measurement of hormone receptors and other tumor markers in breast cancer can provide valuable information for diagnosis, prognosis, and clinical management. The variety of methodologies and the number of potentially useful markers continue to increase. Although most of the work has been performed on tissues, studies performed on ABC material show the feasibility of this approach as well. These encouraging early studies provide a glimpse of an exciting future. The potential exists of applying complex technologies to provide information in multiple dimensions—biochemical, immunologic, and cytopathologic—from cells that are obtained simply by the insertion and aspiration of a small needle.

REFERENCES

1. Agnantis NJ, Petraki C, Markoulatos P, Spandidos DA: Immunohistochemical study of the *ras* oncogene expression in human breast lesions. *Anticancer Res* 6:1157–1160, 1986.

2. Auer G, Eriksson E, Azavedo E, Caspersson T, Wallgren A: Prognostic significance of nuclear DNA content in mammary adenocarcinomas in humans. *Cancer Res* 44:394–396, 1984.

3. Azavedo E, Baral E, Skoog L: Immunohistochemical analysis of estrogen receptors in cells obtained by fine needle aspiration from human mammary carcinomas. *Anticancer Res* 6:263–266, 1986.

4. Bacus S, Flowers JL, Press MF, Bacus JW, McCarty KS Jr: The evaluation of estrogen receptor in primary breast carcinoma by computer-assisted image analysis. *Am J Clin Pathol* 90:233–239, 1988.

5. Bahu RM, Mangkornkanok-Mark M, Albertson D, et al: Detection of alpha-lactalbumin in breast lesions and relationship to estrogen receptors and serum prolactin. *Cancer* 46:1775–1780, 1980.

6. Bailey AJ, Sloane JP, Trickey BS, Ormerod MG: An immunocytochemical study of alpha-lactalbumin in human breast tissue. *J Pathol* 137:13–23, 1982.

7. Barnard NJ, Hall PA, Lemoine NR, Kadar N: Proliferative index in breast carcinoma determined *in situ* by Ki67 immunostaining and its relationship to clinical and pathological variables. *J Pathol* 152:287–295, 1987.

8. Barry JD, Koch TJ, Cohen C, Brigati DJ, Sharkey FE: Correlation of immunohistochemical markers with patient prognosis in breast carcinoma: A quantitative study. *Am J Clin Pathol* 82:582–585, 1984.

9. Beatson GT: On the treatment of inoperable cases of carcinoma of the mamma: Suggestions for a new method of treatment with illustrative cases. *Lancet* 2:104–107, 1896.

10. Benyahia B, Magdelenat H, Zajdela A, Vilcoq JR: Fine needle aspirate estrogen receptor assay in breast tumors. *Bull Cancer (Paris)* 69:456–460, 1982.

11. Bibbo M, Dytch HE, Puls JH, Bartels PH, Wied GL: Clinical applications for an inexpensive, microcomputer-based DNA-cytometry system. *Acta Cytol* 30:372–378, 1986.

12. Bishop HM, Elston CW, Blamey RW, Haybittle JL, Nicholson RI, et al: Relationship of oestrogen-receptor status to survival in breast cancer. *Lancet* 2:283–284, 1979.

13. Bloom HJG, Richardson WW: Histologic grading and prognosis in breast cancer: A study of 1409 cases of which 359 have been followed for 15 years. *Br J Cancer* 11:359–377, 1957.

14. Bridges KG, Keshgegian AA, Kumar HAM, Schiowitz RF, Neal HS: Influence of surgical technique on estrogen and progesterone receptor determinations in breast cancer. *Cancer* 51:2317–2320, 1983.

15. Candlish W, Kerr IB, Simpson HW: Immunocytochemical demonstration and significance of p21 *ras* family oncogene product in benign and malignant breast disease. *J Pathol* 159:163–167, 1986.

16. Cavailles V, Garcia M, Salazar G, et al: Immunodetection of estrogen receptor and 52,000-dalton protein in fine needle aspirates of breast cancer tumors. *J Natl Cancer Inst* 79:245–252, 1987

17. Chamness GC, Mercer WD, McGuire WL: Are histochemical methods for estrogen receptor valid? *J Histochem Cytochem* 28:792–798, 1980.

18. Chess Q, Hajdu SI: The role of immunoperoxidase staining in diagnostic cytology. *Acta Cytol* 30:1–7, 1986.

19. Clair T, Miller WR, Cho-Chung YS: Prognostic significance of the expression of a *ras* protein with a molecular weight of 21,000 by human breast cancer. *Cancer Res* 47:5290–5293, 1987.

20. Clark GM, McGuire WL: Steroid receptors and other prognostic factors in primary breast cancer. *Semin Oncol* 15 (Suppl 1):20–25, 1988.

21. Clayton F, Ordonez NG, Hanssen GM, Hanssen H: Immunoperoxidase localization of lactalbumin in malignant breast neoplasms. *Arch Pathol Lab Med* 106:268–270, 1982.

22. Colvin RB, Preffer FI: New technologies in cell analysis by flow cytometry. *Arch Pathol Lab Med* 111:628–632, 1987.

23. Coombes RC, Berger U, McClelland RA, et al: Prediction of endocrine response in breast cancer by immunocytochemical detection of oestrogen receptors in fine-needle aspirates. *Lancet* 2:701–703, 1987.

24. Crawford DJ, Lope-Pihie A, Cowan S, George WD, Leake RE: Pre-operative determination of oestrogen receptor status in breast cancer by immunocytochemical staining of fine needle aspirates. *Br J Surg* 72:991–993, 1985.

25. Curtin CT, Pertschuk LP, Mitchell V: Histochemical determination of estrogen and progesterone binding in fine needle aspirates of breast cancer: Correlation with conventional biochemical assays. *Acta Cytol* 26:841–846, 1982.

26. DeGoeij TFPM, Bosman FT, Berns EMJJ: Determination of steroid hormone dependency of tumors utilizing tissue sections: Survey of histochemical techniques and their application in surgical pathology. *J Pathol* 149:163–172, 1986.

27. DeSombre ER, Jensen EV: Estrophilin assays in breast cancer: Quantitative features and application to the mastectomy specimen. *Cancer* 46:2783–2788, 1980.

28. DeSombre ER, Thorpe SM, Rose C, et al: Prognostic usefulness of estrogen receptor immunocytochemical assays for human breast cancer. *Cancer Res* 46:4256s–4264s, 1986.

29. Domagala W, Lubinski J, Weber K, Osborn M: Intermediate filament typing of tumor cells in fine needle aspirates by means of monoclonal antibodies. *Acta Cytol* 30:214–224, 1986.

30. Doria MI Jr, Adamec T, Talerman A: Alpha-lactalbumin in "common" epithelial tumors of the ovary: An immunohistochemical study. *Am J Clin Pathol* 87:752–756, 1987.

31. Dressler LG, Seamer LC, Owens MA, Clark GM, McQuire WL: DNA flow cytometry and prognostic factors in 1331 frozen breast cancer specimens. *Cancer* 61:420–427, 1988.

32. Drier JK, Swanson PE, Cherwitz DL, Wick MR: S-100 protein immunoreactivity in poorly-differentiated carcinomas: Immunohistochemical comparison with malignant melanoma. *Arch Pathol Lab Med* 111:444–452, 1987.

33. Earl M: Cell collection from fine needle aspirates for estrogen receptor immunocytochemical assay. *Acta Cytol* 31:377–378, 1987.

34. Ellis IO, Bell J, Todd JM, et al: Evaluation of immunoreactivity with monoclonal antibody NCRC 11 in breast carcinoma. *Br J Cancer* 56:295–299, 1987.

35. Eusebi V, Millis RR, Cattani MG, Bussolati G, Azzopardi JG: Apocrine carcinoma of the breast: A morphologic and immunocytochemical study. *Am J Pathol* 123:532–541, 1986.

36. Fisher B, Redmond C, Fisher ER, et al: Relative worth of estrogen or progesterone receptor and pathologic characteristics of differentiation as indicators of prognosis in node negative breast cancer patients: Findings from National Surgical Adjuvant Breast and Bowel Project Protocol B-06. *J Clin Oncol* 6:1076–1087, 1988.

37. Flowers JL, Burton GV, Cox EB, et al: Use of monoclonal antiestrogen receptor antibody to evaluate estrogen receptor content in fine needle aspiration breast biopsies. *Ann Surg* 203:250–254, 1986.

38. Flowers J, Burton G, Geisinger K, et al: Fine needle aspiration biopsy: Immunohistochemical analysis of ER and PR versus clinical response. *Lab Invest* 56:24A, 1987.

39. Franklin WA: Tissue binding of lectins in disorders of the breast. *Cancer* 51:295–300, 1983.

40. Gal R, Gukovsky-Oren S, Lehman JM, Schwartz P, Kessler E: Cytodiagnosis of a spindle-cell tumor of the breast using antisera to epithelial membrane antigen. *Acta Cytol* 31:317–321, 1987.

41. Garrett CT: Oncogenes. *Clin Chim Acta* 156:1–40, 1986.

42. Gerdes J, Pickartz H, Brotherton J, et al: Growth factions and estrogen receptors in human breast cancers as determined *in situ* with monoclonal antibodies. *Am J Pathol* 129:486–492, 1987.

43. Ghosh AK, Moore M, Harris M: Immunohistochemical detection of *ras* oncogene p21 product in benign and malignant mammary tissue in man. *J Clin Pathol* 39:428–434, 1986.

44. Greene GL, Sobel NB, King WJ, Jensen EV: Immunochemical studies of estrogen receptors. *J Steroid Biochem* 20:51–56, 1984.

45. Greenwalt DE, Johnson VG, Kuhajda FP, Eggleston JC, Mather IH: Localization of a membrane glycoprotein in benign fibrocystic disease and infiltrating duct carcinomas of the human breast with the use of a monoclonal antibody to guinea pig milk fat globule membrane. *Am J Pathol* 118:351–359, 1985.

46. Gunduz N, Zheng S, Fisher B: Fluoresceinated estrone binding by cells from human breast cancers obtained by needle aspiration. *Cancer* 52:1251–1256, 1983.

47. Gupta RK, Wakefield SJ, Holloway LJ, Simpson JS: Immunocytochemical and ultra-structural study of the rare osteoclast-type carcinoma of the breast in a fine needle aspirate. *Acta Cytol* 32:79–82, 1988.

48. Guzman J, Costabel V, Bross KJ, et al: The value of the immunoperoxidase slide assay in the diagnosis of malignant pleural effusions in breast cancer. *Acta Cytol* 32:188–192, 1988.

49. Hahnel R, Woodings T, Vivian AB: Prognostic value of estrogen receptors in primary breast cancer. *Cancer* 44:671–675, 1979.

50. Hawkins RA, Sangster K, Krajewski A: Histochemical detection of oestrogen receptors in breast carcinoma: A successful technique. *Br J Cancer* 53:407–410, 1986.

51. Helin HJ, Helle MJ, Helin ML, Isola JJ: Immunocytochemical detection of estrogen and progesterone receptors in 124 human breast cancers. *Am J Clin Pathol* 90:137–142, 1988.

52. Heuson JC, Longeval E, Mattheiem WH, et al: Significance of quantitative assessment of estrogen receptors for endocrine therapy in advanced breast cancer. *Cancer* 39:1971–1977, 1977.

53. Horne CHW, Reid IN, Milne GD: Prognostic significance of inappropriate production of pregnancy proteins by breast cancers. *Lancet* 2:279–282, 1976.

54. Horwitz KB, McGuire WL, Pearson OH, Segaloff A: Predicting response to endocrine therapy in human breast cancer: A hypothesis. *Science* 189:726–727, 1975.

55. Jensen EV: Historical perspective. *Cancer* 46:2759–2761, 1980.

56. Jensen EV: Intracellular localization of estrogen receptors: Implications for interaction mechanism. *Lab Invest* 51:487–488, 1984.

57. Jensen EV, DeSombre ER: The diagnostic implications of steroid binding in malignant tissues. *Adv Clin Chem* 19:57–89, 1977.

58. Johnston WW, Szpak CA, Lottich SC, Thor A, Schlom J: Use of a monoclonal antibody (B72.3) as a novel immunohistochemical adjunct for the diagnosis of carcinoma in fine needle aspiration biopsy specimens. *Hum Pathol* 17:501–513, 1986.

59. Johnston WW, Szpak CA, Lottich SC, Thor A, Schlom J: Use of a monoclonal antibody (B72.3) as an immunocytochemical adjunct to diagnosis of adenocarcinoma in human effusions. *Cancer Res* 45:1894–1900, 1985.

60. Jonat W, Maass H, Stegner HE: Immunohistochemical measurement of estrogen receptors in breast cancer tissue samples. *Cancer Res* 46:4296s–4298s, 1986.

61. Keshgegian AA: ABCs of immunocytochemistry, in Kline TS: *Handbook of Fine Needle Aspiration Biopsy Cytology,* ed 2. New York, Churchill Livingstone, 1988, pp 419–431.

62. Keshgegian AA: Immunocytochemistry, in Kline TS: *Guides to Clinical Aspiration Biopsy: Prostate.* New York, Igaku-Shoin, 1985, pp 115–125.

63. Keshgegian AA, Inverso K, Kline TS: Determination of estrogen receptor by monoclonal antireceptor antibody in aspiration biopsy cytology from breast carcinoma. *Am J Clin Pathol* 89:24–29, 1988.

64. Keshgegian AA, Wheeler JE: Estrogen receptor protein in malignant carcinoid tumor: A report of 2 cases. *Cancer* 45:293–296, 1980.

65. Kiang DT, Kennedy BJ: Estrogen receptor assay in the differential diagnosis of adeno-carcinomas. *JAMA* 238:32–34, 1977.

66. King WJ, DeSombre ER, Jensen EV, Greene GL: Comparison of immunocytochemical and steroid-binding assays for estrogen receptor in human breast tumors. *Cancer Res* 45:293–304, 1985.

67. King WJ, Greene GL: Monoclonal antibodies localize oestrogen receptor in the nuclei of target cells. *Nature* 307:745–747, 1984.

68. Kinsel L, Flowers J, Cox E, et al: Use of a monoclonal antiprogesterone receptor antibody to complement immunohistochemical evaluation of ER in breast tumors. *Lab Invest* 56:38A, 1987.

69. Knight WA, Livingston RB, Gregory EJ, McGuire WL: Estrogen receptor as an independent prognostic indicator for early recurrence in breast cancer. *Cancer Res* 37:4669–4671, 1977.

70. Kuhajda FP, Eggleston JC: Pregnancy associated plasma protein A: A clinically significant predictor of early recurrence in stage I breast carcinoma is independent of estrogen receptor status. *Am J Pathol* 121:342–348, 1985.

71. Kuhajda FP, Offutt LE, Mendelsohn G: The distribution of carcinoembryonic antigen in breast carcinoma: Diagnostic and prognostic implications. *Cancer* 52:1257–1264, 1983.

72. Kurtin PJ, Pinkus GS: Leukocyte common antigen—a diagnostic discriminant between hematopoietic and nonhematopoietic neoplasms in paraffin sections using monoclonal antibodies: Correlation with immunologic studies and ultrastructural localization. *Hum Pathol* 16:353–364, 1985.

73. Lampertico P, Stagni F: Cytology and hormonal receptors in breast cancer. *Diagn Cytopathol* 2:17–23, 1986.

74. Lee AK, DeLellis RA, Rosen PP, et al: ABH blood group isoantigen expression in breast carcinomas—an immunohistochemical evaluation using monoclonal antibodies. *Am J Clin Pathol* 83:308–319, 1985.

75. Lee AK, Rosen PP, DeLellis RA, et al: Tumor marker expression in breast carcinomas and relationship to prognosis: An immunohistochemical study. *Am J Clin Pathol* 84:687–696, 1985.

76. Lee AK, Tallberg K, DeLillis RA, et al: Alpha-lactalbumin as an immunohistochemical marker for metastatic breast carcinomas. *Am J Surg Pathol* 8:93–100, 1984.

77. Lee SH: Cytochemical study of estrogen receptor in human mammary cancer. *Am J Clin Pathol* 70:197–203, 1978.

78. Levack PA, Mullen P, Anderson TJ, Miller WR, Forrest APM: DNA analysis of breast tumor fine needle aspirates using flow cytometry. *Br J Cancer* 56:643–646, 1987.

79. Lloyd RV, Foley J, Judd WJ: Peanut lectin agglutinin and alpha-lactalbumin: Binding and immunohistochemical localization in breast tissues. *Arch Pathol Lab Med* 108:392–395, 1984.

80. Lozowski MS, Mishriki Y, Chao S, et al: Estrogen receptor determination in fine needle aspirates of the breast: Correlation with histologic grade and comparison with biochemical analysis. *Acta Cytol* 31:557–562, 1987.

81. Lundy J, Kline TS, Lozowski M, Chao S: Immunoperoxidase studies by monoclonal antibody B72.3 applied to breast aspirates: Diagnostic considerations. *Diagn Cytopathol* 4:95–98, 1988.

82. Lundy J, Lozowski M, Mishriki Y: Monoclonal antibody B72.3 as a diagnostic adjunct in fine needle aspirates of breast masses. *Ann Surg* 203:399–402, 1986.

83. McCarty KS Jr, Hiatt KB, Budwit DA, et al: Clinical response to hormone therapy correlated with estrogen receptor analysis: Biochemical vs. histochemical methods. *Arch Pathol Lab Med* 108:24–26, 1984.

84. McCarty KS Jr, Miller LS, Cox EB, Konrath J, McCarty KS Sr: Estrogen receptor analysis: correlation of biochemical and immunohistochemical methods using monoclonal antireceptor antibodies. *Arch Pathol Lab Med* 109:716–721, 1985.

85. McCarty KS Jr, Szabo E, Flowers JL, et al: Use of a monoclonal anti-estrogen receptor antibody in the immunohistochemical evaluation of human tumors. *Cancer Res* 46:4244s–4248s, 1986.

86. McClelland RA, Berger U, Miller LS, Powles TJ, Coombes RC: Immunocytochemical assay for estrogen receptor in patients with breast cancer: Relationship to a biochemical assay and to outcome of therapy. *J Clin Oncol* 4:1171–1176, 1986.

87. McClelland RA, Berger U, Wilson P, et al: Presurgical determination of estrogen receptor status using immunocytochemically stained fine needle aspirate smears in patients with breast cancer. *Cancer Res* 47:6118–6122, 1987.

88. McGee JO'D, Woods JC, Ashall F, Bramwell ME, Harris H: A new marker for human cancer cells. 2. Immunohistochemical detection of the Ca antigen in human tissues with the Cal antibody. *Lancet* 2:7–10, 1982.

89. McGuire WL, Dressler LG: Emerging impact of flow cytometry in predicting recurrence and survival in breast cancer patients. *J Natl Cancer Inst* 75:405–410, 1985.

90. Magdelenat H, Laine-Bidron C, Merle S, Zajdela A: Estrogen and progestin receptor assay in fine needle aspirates of breast cancer: methodological aspects. *Eur J Cancer Clin Oncol* 23:425–431, 1987.

91. Magdelenat H, Merle S, Zajdela A: Enzyme immunoassay of estrogen receptors in fine needle aspirates of breast tumors. *Cancer Res* 46:4265s–4167s, 1986.

92. Mansour EG, Hastert M, Park CH, Koehler KA, Petrelli M: Tissue and plasma carcinoembryonic antigen in early breast cancer: A prognostic factor. *Cancer* 51:1243–1248, 1983.

93. Martin SE, Moshiri S, Thor A, et al: Identification of adenocarcinoma in cytospin preparations of effusions using monoclonal antibody B72.3. *Am J Clin Pathol* 86:10–18, 1986.

94. Mazoujian G, Pinkus GS, Davis S, Haagensen DE Jr: Immunohistochemistry of a gross cystic disease fluid protein (GCDFP-15) of the breast: A marker of apocrine epithelium and breast carcinomas with apocrine features. *Am J Pathol* 110:105–112, 1983.

95. Mercer WD, Lippman ME, Wahl TM, et al: The use of immunocytochemical techniques for the detection of steroid hormones in breast cancer cells. *Cancer* 46:2859–2868, 1980.

96. Merle S, Zajdela A, Magdelenat H: Progesterone-receptor assay in fine needle aspirates of breast tumors. *Acta Cytol* 29:496–498, 1985.

97. Murthy L, Kapila K, Verma K: Immunoperoxidase detection of carcinoembryonic antigen in fine needle aspirates of breast carcinoma: Correlation with studies in tissue sections. *Acta Cytol* 32:60–62, 1988.

98. Nakajima T, Kameya T, Watanabe S, et al: An immunoperoxidase study of S-100 protein distribution in normal and neoplastic tissues. *Am J Surg Pathol* 6:715–727, 1982.

99. Nesland JM, Holm R, Johannessen JV, Goule VE: Neuron specific enolase immunostaining in the diagnosis of breast carcinomas with neuroendocrine differentiation: Its usefulness and limitations. *J Pathol* 148:35–43, 1986.

100. Nuti M, Teramoto YA, Mariani-Constantini R, et al: A monoclonal antibody (B72.3) defines patterns of distribution of a novel tumor-associated antigen in human mammary carcinoma cell populations. *Int J Cancer* 29:539–545, 1982.

101. Osborne CK: Heterogeneity in hormone receptor status in primary and metastatic breast cancer. *Semin Oncol* 12:317–326, 1985.

102. Osborne CK, Yochmowitz MG, Knight WA, McGuire WL: The value of estrogen and progesterone receptors in the treatment of breast cancer. *Cancer* 46:2884–2888, 1980.

103. Oxenhandler RW, McCune R, Subtelney A, Truelove C, Tyrer HW: Flow cytometric determination of estrogen receptors in intact cells. *Cancer Res* 44:2516–2523, 1984.

104. Ozello L, de Rosa CM, Konrath JG, Yeager JL, Miller LS: Detection of estrophilin in frozen sections of breast cancers using an estrogen receptor immunocytochemical assay. *Cancer Res* 46:4303s–4307s, 1986.

105. Panko WB, Mattioli CA, Wheeler TM: Lack of correlation of a histochemical method for estrogen receptor analysis with the biochemical assay results. *Cancer* 49:2148–2152, 1982.

106. Perrot-Applanat M, Groyer-Picard M-T, Lorenzo F, et al: Immunocytochemical study with monoclonal antibodies to progesterone receptor in human breast tumors. *Cancer Res* 47:2652–2661, 1987.

107. Pertschuk LP, Eisenberg KB, Carter AC, Feldman JG: Immunohistologic localization of estrogen receptors in breast cancer with monoclonal antibodies: Correlation with biochemistry and clinical endocrine response. *Cancer* 55:1513–1518, 1985.

108. Pertschuk LP, Feldman JG, Eisenberg KB, et al: Immunocytochemical detection of progesterone receptor in breast cancer with monoclonal antibody: Relation to biochemical assay, disease-free survival and clinial endocrine response. *Cancer* 62:342–349, 1988.

109. Pertschuk LP, Gaetjens E, Carter AC, et al: Histochemistry of steroid receptors: An overview. *Ann Clin Lab Sci* 9:219–224, 1979.

110. Pichon M-F, Pallud C, Brunet M, Milgrom E: Relationship of presence of progesterone receptors to prognosis in early breast cancer. *Cancer Res* 40:3357–3360, 1980.

111. Poulsen HS, Schultz H, Bichel P: Oestrogen-receptor determinations on fine-needle aspirates from malignant tumours of the breast. *Eur J Cancer* 15:1431–1438, 1979.

112. Raam S, Gelman R, Cohen JL, et al: Estrogen receptor assay: Interlaboratory and intralaboratory variations in the measurement of receptors using dextran-coated charcoal technique: A study sponsored by E.C.O.G. *Eur J Cancer* 17:643–649, 1981.

113. Ramaekers F, Haag D, Jap P, Vooijs PG: Immunochemical demonstration of keratin and vimentin in cytologic aspirates. *Acta Cytol* 28:385–392, 1984.

114. Rasmussen BB, Pederson BV, Thorpe SM, et al: Prognostic value of surface antigens in primary human breast carcinomas, detected by monoclonal antibodies. *Cancer Res* 45:1424–1427, 1985.

115. Reiner A, Reiner G, Spona J, et al: Estrogen receptor immunocytochemistry for preoperative determination of estrogen receptor status on fine-needle aspirates of breast cancer. *Am J Clin Pathol* 88:399–404, 1987.

116. Reiner A, Spona J, Reiner G, et al: Estrogen receptor analysis on biopsies and fine-needle aspirates from human breast carcinoma: Correlation of biochemical and immunohistochemical methods using monoclonal antireceptor antiboides. *Am J Pathol* 125:443–449, 1986.

117. Sainsbury JRC, Needham GK, Farndon JR, Malcolm AJ, Harris AL: Epidermal growth-factor receptor status as predictor of early recurrence of and death from breast cancer. *Lancet* 1:1398–1402, 1987.

118. Scheres HME, de Goeij AFPM, Rousch MJM, et al: Quantification of oestrogen recep-

tors in breast cancer: Radiochemical assays on cytosols and cryostat sections compared with semiquantitative immunocytochemical analysis. *J Clin Pathol* 41:623–632, 1988.

119. Sheikh FA, Tinkoff GH, Kline TS, Neal HS: Final diagnosis by fine-needle aspiration biopsy for definitive operation in breast cancer. *Am J Surg* 154:470–474, 1987.

120. Shousha S, Lyssiotis T, Godfrey VM, Scheuer PJ: Carcinoembryonic antigen in breast-cancer tissue: A useful prognostic indicator. *Br Med J* 1:777–779, 1979.

121. Silfversward C, Gustafsson J-A, Gustafsson SA, et al: Estrogen receptor analysis on fine needle aspirates and on histologic biopsies from human breast cancer. *Eur J Cancer* 16:1351–1357, 1980.

122. Silfversward C, Humla S: Estrogen receptor analysis on needle aspirates from human mammary carcinoma. *Acta Cytol* 24:54–57, 1980.

123. Silfversward C, Wallgren A, Nordenskjold B, Humla S: Estrogen receptor analysis on fine needle aspirates from human breast carcinoma. *Recent Results Cancer Res* 91:41–44, 1984.

124. Slamon DJ, Clark GM, Wong SG, et al: Human breast cancer: Correlation of relapse and survival with amplification of the HER-2/*neu* oncogene. *Science* 235:177–182, 1987.

125. Stanford JL, Szklo M, Brinton LA: Estrogen receptors and breast cancer. *Epidemiol Rev* 8:42–59, 1986.

126. Szpak CA, Johnston WW, Lottich SC, et al: Patterns of reactivity of four novel mono-clonal antibodies (B72.3, DF3, B1.1, and B6.2) with cells in human malignant and benign effusions. *Acta Cytol* 28:356–367, 1984.

127. Tamura H, Raam S, Nemeth E, et al: Immunohistochemical detection of estrogen receptors in human breast carcinoma using antireceptor antibodies: Its application to cytologic material. *Lab Invest* 46:82A, 1982.

128. Tapia FJ, Polak JM, Barbosa AJA, et al: Neuron-specific enolase is produced by neuro-endocrine tumors. *Lancet* 1:808–811, 1981.

129. Theillet C, Lidereau R, Escot C, et al: Loss of a c-H-*ras*-1 allele and aggressive human primary breast carcinomas. *Cancer Res* 46:4776–4781, 1986.

130. Thor A, Ohuchi N, Hand PH, et al: *ras* Gene alterations and enhanced levels of *ras* p21 expression in a spectrum of benign and malignant human mammary tissues. *Lab Invest* 55:603–615, 1986.

131. Thor A, Ohuchi N, Szpak CA, Johnston WW, Schlom J: Distribution of oncofetal antigen tumor-associated glycoprotein-72 defined by monoclonal antibody B72.3. *Cancer Res* 46:3118–3124, 1986.

132. Travis WD, Wold LE: Immunoperoxidase staining of fine needle aspiration specimens previously stained by the Papanicolaou technique. *Acta Cytol* 31:517–520, 1987.

133. Van NT, Raber M, Barrows GH, Barlogie B: Estrogen receptor analysis by flow cytometry. *Science* 224:876–879, 1984.

134. Venter DJ, Tuzi NL, Kumar S, Gullick WJ: Overexpression of the c-*erb*B-2 oncoprotein in human breast carcinomas: Immunohistological assessment correlates with gene amplification. *Lancet* 2:69–72, 1987.

135. Wachner R, Wittekind C, von Kleist S: Immunohistological localization of B-HCG in breast carcinomas. *Eur J Cancer Clin Oncol* 20:679–684, 1984.

136. Walker RA: Biological markers in human breast carcinoma. *J Pathol* 137:109–117, 1982.

137. Walker RA: The demonstration of alpha-lactalbumin in human breast carcinomas. *J Pathol* 129:37–42, 1979.

138. Walts AE, Said JW: Specific tumor markers in diagnostic cytology: Immunoperoxidase studies of carcinoembryonic antigen, lysozyme, and other tissue antigens in effusions, washes and aspirates. *Acta Cytol* 27:408–416, 1983.

139. Weintraub J, Weintraub D, Redard M, Vassilakos P: Evaluation of estrogen receptors on fine-needle aspiration biopsy specimens from breast tumors. *Cancer* 60:1163–1172, 1987.

140. Wilander E, Pahlman S, Sallstrom J, Lindgren A: Neuron-specific enolase expression and neuroendocrine differentiation in carcinomas of the breast. *Arch Pathol Lab Med* 111:830–832, 1987.

141. Wittliff JL: Steroid-hormone receptors in breast cancer. *Cancer* 53:630–643, 1984.

142. Wrba F, Ritzinger E, Reiner A, Holzner JH: Transferrin receptor expression in breast carcinoma and its possible relationship to prognosis: An immunohistochemical study. *Virchows Arch (Pathol Anat)* 410:69–73, 1986.

12

Future Considerations

HIGH-RISK LESIONS

Pathology

Introduction

These lesions of the breast, often associated with fibrocystic alterations, encompass lobular and ductal proliferative and neoplastic disease. This spectrum of mammary disease includes ductal hyperplasia and atypical hyperplasia; lobular atypical hyperplasia and in situ carcinoma; and intraductal (in situ) carcinoma. The incidence is continually increasing because while some lesions are detected by palpation, the majority are now discovered in asymptomatic patients by screening mammography.

Collectively, this area of breast disease is the most complex for the radiologist, pathologist, and clinician (see "The Surgeon and NAB" in Chapter 8, and Chapter 10). Due to the wide range of histopathologic alterations, some lesions are difficult to delineate, even by the experienced surgical pathologist. Many are indicators of increased risk for the eventual development of invasive carcinoma. Therefore, prediction of their biologic behavior becomes the perplexing task of the clinician who must counsel the patient and present options in management.

Most of these lesions arise in the terminal ductal-lobular unit (TDLU). According to Wellings et al.,[20] the lobular acini coalesce and expand, leading to few but markedly enlarged ductules. This lobular concept is referred to as "unfolding." Formerly, the transformed ductular spaces were mistaken for larger ducts. Wellings et al.[20] postulated that the initial change was an atypical lobule which then progressed either to intraductal or to in situ lobular carcinoma by diverging pathways. Azzopardi,[1] however, believed that carcinoma arises de novo from normal structures, undergoing a borderline change prior to the development of frank malignant tumor.

Ductal Hyperplasia

Epithelial hyperplasia is a condition involving an increase in the usual two layers of cells lining the ductule.[13] In mild hyperplasia there is no more than a four-cell thickness; in moderate hyperplasia, somewhat more; in florid hyperplasia, swirls of cells may obliterate the lumen or leave a few slitted central or peripheral spaces. The cells usually are rounded, with finely granular chromatin, but display variably sized nuclei, nucleoli, and some mitotic activity. Mild and moderate hyperplasia carry no enhanced risk of carcinoma, but florid hyperplasia may indicate 1.5 to 2 times the risk of the general population.[13]

Atypical Ductal Hyperplasia

Atypical ductal hyperplasia has some features of in situ carcinoma. Generally, however, there is preservation of irregular luminal slits. Although the peripheral portions of the ductule often are partially lined by the normal columnar layer, centrally the cell population may be monomorphic, with marked nuclear irregularity and hyperchromasia. A diagnosis of benignity is warranted when only a single ductule is completely involved by a lesion indistinguishable from that of in situ carcinoma.[13]

The incidence of atypical hyperplasia is about 2 percent. It is rarely found before the age of 35 and rises to about 4 percent in the 35- to 55-year age group.[13] In these patients, the risk of the later development of cancer is about 4 times that of the general population, while for those with a familial history of carcinoma it is increased 8 to 10 times.[13]

In-Situ Lobular Carcinoma

This neoplasm, first described by Foote and Stewart[4] in 1941, is recognized as a special carcinoma, arising in and confined to the lobular acini, multicentric, bilateral, and bearing some relationship to invasive carcinoma. Most lesions are grossly inapparent and have been found fortuitously in otherwise benign breast biopsy specimens with an incidence of 0.8 to 3.8 percent.[5] Today the frequency is greater because of mammographic screening, with the discovery of associated finely stippled microcalcifications.[6] The majority of these lesions occur in premenopausal women,[5] but 10 to 25 percent are reported in later life.[15] Most are found in the upper outer quadrant and almost half within 5.0 cm of the nipple.[10] Contralateral blind biopsies in this area, as well as mirror-image biopsy, often disclose a second neoplasm.[6]

Microscopically, only one or two lobules may be affected, or there may be diffuse disease. The characteristic finding within the acini is a proliferation of cells, resulting in luminal disappearance and acinar distention. Two types of tumor cells have been described. The more common one consists of small, bland cells with pale, indistinct cytoplasm and oval, hyperchromatic nuclei; less frequently, the cells become anaplastic. Some mitoses may be apparent, and necrosis is absent.[4,11] This lesion is differentiated from atypical lobular hyperplasia in that more than half of the acini within the lobule must be involved in the in situ carcinoma.[14]

In situ lobular carcinoma presents a distinct clinical problem. Lattes[11] preferred the term "lobular neoplasia," commenting that it was "a multifocal microscopic entity of uncertain and controversial clinical significance, not definitely irreversible nor leading to invasive carcinoma." Haagensen et al.[5] stressed that lobular neoplasia is a high-risk marker. McDivitt et al.,[12] after follow-up studies of 50 women treated chiefly by local excision, reported that infiltrating carcinoma developed in 8 percent after 5 years, 15 percent after 10 years, 27 percent after 15 years, and 35 percent after 20 years; almost half of the carcinomas were found in the contralateral breast. The authors estimated that by 23 years following surgery, the cumulative risk was greater than 50 percent. A subsequent 24-year study of 99 patients revealed 39 carcinomas in 32 patients and a risk factor nine times greater than that of the general population.[16] While the only preventive therapy is bilateral mastectomy, an acceptable alternative is contralateral biopsy with patient counseling regarding the risk factor and lifetime follow-up examinations.[5,11]

Intraductal Carcinoma

Intraductal carcinoma (in situ ductal carcinoma) of the breast, first clinically recognized in 1932 by Broders,[2] is a neoplasm in which the malignant cells are confined to a preexisting ductal structure. The tumor is discovered by a mass, nipple discharge, or mammographic small, clustered microcalcifications. The patients average 50 years of age, a few years lower than the average age for the development of infiltrating ductal carcinoma. In most series the incidence is between 2 and 3 percent,[17] but it has increased because of mammographic detection; in one series of selected patients, it was 18 percent.[19]

Histologically, these lesions include solid, cribriform, papillary, comedo, and mixed patterns. When the entire duct is expanded by tumor cells, the solid type is formed. With central necrosis, the comedo type is diagnosed. The cribriform type is composed of tumor cells oriented around multiple rounded lumens rather than the duct. Small papillary formations without central vascular cores lead to the diagnosis of micropapillary tumor. The mixed variety consists of combinations of the various elements. The malignant epithelium is composed of monomorphic, sometimes markedly anaplastic cells with enlarged, hyperchromatic nuclei, numerous mitoses, and, generally, accompanying necrosis.

The lesions are often multifocal and multicentric. Multicentricity has been demonstrated in 32 to 55 percent of mastectomy specimens.[9,19] Recurrence has been ascribed to this multicentricity and is the basis for treatment by mastectomy. Fisher et al.[3] suggested that similar beneficial results could be achieved by lumpectomy and postoperative irradiation. Because of the low incidence of axillary lymph node metastases,[18] axillary dissection may be an unnecessary procedure.

ABC

Introduction

More and more of these lesions are being sampled by NAB. While some specimens are obtained from palpable masses, most are taken from clinically occult lesions. The latter are procured serendipitously, or with the scouting needle (see Chapter 2), or with image localization (see Chapter 10).

Recognition of these aspirated cells may be relatively easy or may require intense scrutiny of the slide contents. In the former situation, the cells must be distinguished from those of infiltrating carcinoma. This problem is more common in specimens from nonpalpable masses acquired either by the scouting needle or by mammographic localization. With palpable masses the clinical situation, as well as the number of abnormal cells, generally provide significant landmarks.

Microcalcifications may be seen in the ABC from all lesions. These are nonspecific, however, and are found not only with infiltrating carcinomas and high-risk lesions but also with fibrocystic change alone (see Figs. 4-4, 6-6, and 6-17). Nonetheless, their presence in aspirates from occult tumors may signify that representative material has been retrieved.

Atypical Ductal Hyperplasia

This lesion must be included in the differential diagnosis when there are small numbers of abnormal cells. Although the majority of the cells are indicative of fibrocystic change, among the benign groups are a few cells clustered in atypical patterns. Relatively loosely arranged, nonpolarized, small groups may be seen. There may be a few papillae. The individual cells are modest in size, with indistinctly bounded cytoplasm. The nuclei may be relatively uniform, with finely granular chromatin, or may display anisonucleosis and rare macronucleoli (Fig. 12.1).

The architectural and cellular alterations associated with atypical hyperplasia are occasionally seen with fibrocystic change. Cells from ductal hyperplasia may also reveal loosely clustered cells in unusual patterns (Fig. 12.2) (see Table 12.1 and the sections on "Ductal Hyperplasia" and "Interpretative Traps," in Chapter 4). Currently, all of these cases need tissue biopsy. Perhaps in the future a monoclonal antibody such as B72.3 can be used to distinguish the two lesions. From our series of suspicious aspirates to which MAb B72.3 was applied,[8] there was one case of atypical ductal hyperplasia from a patient with an abnormal mammogram but no mass. The cells, obtained by the scouting needle, reacted positively to the antibody (Plate 2-3).

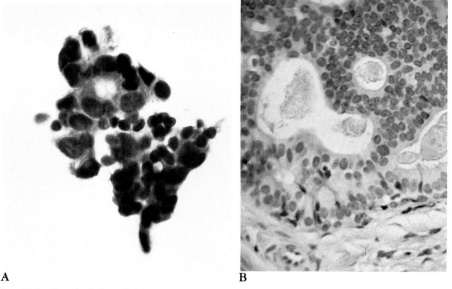

A   B

Fig. 12.1. Atypical ductal hyperplasia. **A.** ABC. Note the configuration of the group. Papanicolaou preparation ($\times 500$). **B.** Tissue section. Hematoxylin and eosin preparation ($\times 300$).

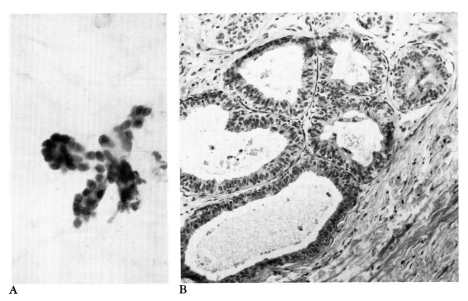

A   B

Fig. 12.2. Ductal hyperplasia, false-suspicious interpretation. **A.** ABC. Note the atypical architecture. Papanicolaou preparation (× 300). **B.** Tissue section. Hematoxylin and eosin preparation (× 125).

In-Situ Lobular Carcinoma

Due to associated fibrocystic change, the ABC from the in situ neoplasm often displays a number of benign cells. The tumor cells, sometimes in focally cellular areas on the slide, form moderate and small-sized groups with some degree of dyshesion. The individual small cells have large nuclei and cytoplasmic rims or wispy, ill-defined cytoplasm. The nuclear membranes may be minimally thickened and irregular, and macronucleoli are not unusual (Fig. 12.3; see Table 12.1). The ABC resembles that from a desmoplastic infiltrating lobular carcinoma and, in our experience, has been interpreted as suggestive of that lesion. Of our recent 25 suspicious aspirates, there was reactivity to MAb B72.3 in one of the three cases of in situ lobular carcinoma[8] (see Plate 2.4).

Intraductal Carcinoma

The ABC from this lesion may have most of the criteria of malignancy. The abnormal cells, however, may be sparse, and there may be some polymorphism due to the presence of benign ductal cells.

The types of cells that are aspirated depend upon the type of intraductal carcinoma. From the comedocarcinoma, a small amount of hemorrhagic fluid may be withdrawn. The modestly cellular ABC consists of dyshesive groups and isolated cells. The cells measure up to 30 μm in diameter, with ill-defined sometimes abundant, orangeophilic cytoplasm and large, irregular, hyperchromatic nuclei[7] (Fig. 12.4). They bear some resemblance to malignant squamous cells. From solid tumors, the cells resemble those of infiltrating ductal carcinoma. They may appear in dyshesive aggregates, in groups of two to five, or, rarely, isolated. They may be

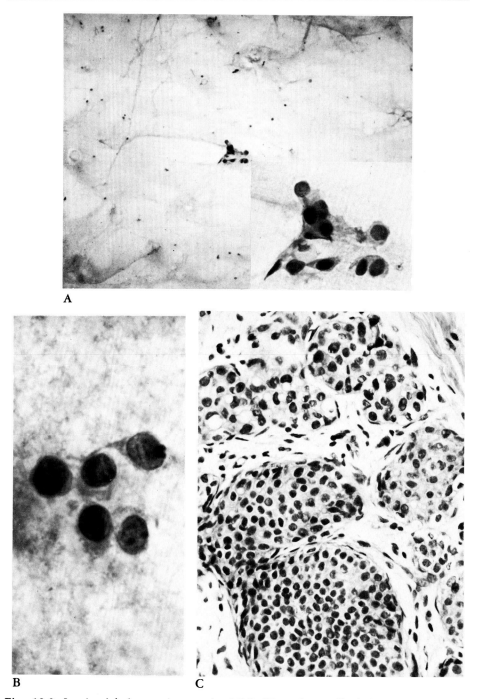

Fig. 12.3. In situ lobular carcinoma. **A.** ABC. Note the small, dyshesive cell group. Papanicolaou preparation (×125). Insert: ABC, higher magnification. Papanicolaou preparation (×500). **B.** ABC. Note the cells with large nuclei and cytoplasmic rims. Papanicolaou preparation (×1250). **C.** Tissue section. Hematoxylin and eosin preparation (×300).

TABLE 12.1 High-risk Lesions: Comparative Cytomorphology

	Atypical Hyperplasia	*In Situ Lobular Carcinoma*	*Intraductal Carcinoma*
Pattern			
Cellularity	−	±	+
Dyshesion	−	+	+
Monomorphism	−	−	±
Nuclear changes*			
Membrane irregularity	±	±	+
Macronucleoli	±	+	+
Special features:	Architectural abnormalities	Similarity to desmoplastic lobular carcinoma	Squamoid cells (comedo-carcinoma)

* All may show anisonucleosis.

fewer in number, however, than those from the infiltrating type. The cribriform pattern is reflected by relatively cohesive, large or small groups with round lumens. There are often a few dyshesive clusters and isolated cells (Fig. 12.5). One specimen procured by the scouting needle from the single intraductal carcinoma in our series displayed positivity to MAb B72.3[8] (see Plate 2.5, Table 12.1).

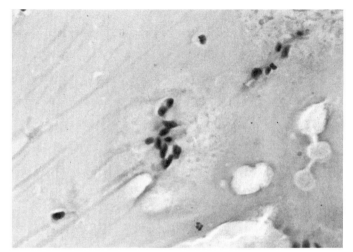

A

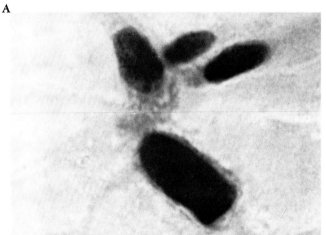

B

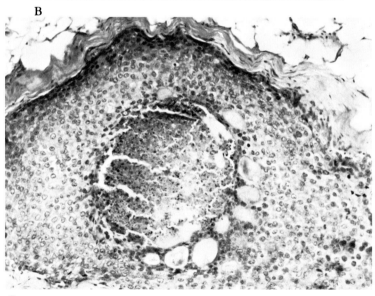

C

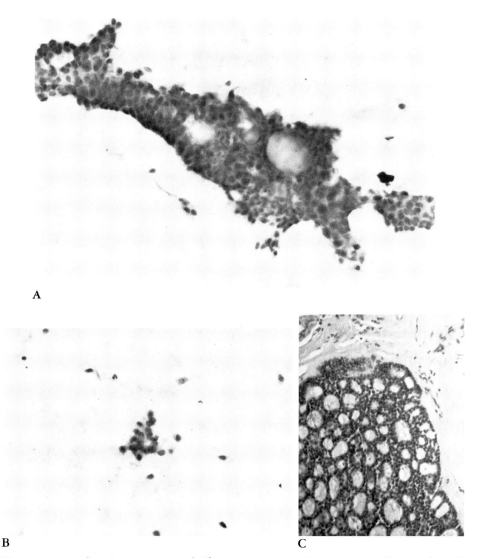

A

B   C

Fig. 12.5. Intraductal carcinoma, cribriform type. **A, B.** ABC. Note the large and small groups with round lumens. Papanicolaou preparations (× 300). **C.** Tissue section. Hematoxylin and eosin preparation (× 125).

Fig. 12.4. Comedocarcinoma. **A.** ABC. Note the dyshesive groups and isolated large cells. Papanicolaou preparation (× 300). **B.** ABC. Note the cells with large, hyperchromatic nuclei Papanicolaou preparation (× 1250). **C.** Tissue section. Hematoxylin and eosin preparation (× 125).

DNA DISTRIBUTION
IN BREAST CARCINOMA:
APPLICATION OF CYTOMETRIC
MEASUREMENTS TO ABC

Sally Rosen, M.D.

Introduction

Investigations of the DNA distribution of human tumors, including breast carcinoma, have suggested that there is a correlation between DNA ploidy levels and patient prognosis.[21,24,34] Current interest has focused on the clinical application of cytometric techniques to the management of the patient with breast cancer.[29,32,33,43]

Methods

Cellular DNA content can be measured with microscope-based cytophotometry or flow cytometry, using a variety of tissue and cytology samples. While both methods yield comparable results for DNA distribution,[22] each has distinct advantages and disadvantages. Either method may be applied to the study of ABC.[23,35,39,44]

Cytophotometry is a microscope-based technique which uses fluorescence measurements of single cells to produce a histogram of DNA distribution (Figs. 12.6, 12.7). Measurements can be performed on fresh imprints or aspirates and on

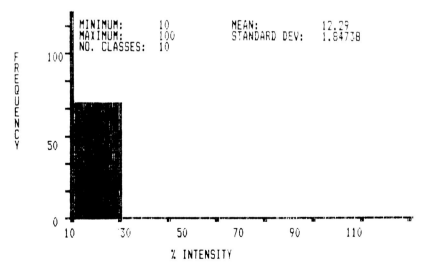

Fig. 12.6. Histogram of peripheral blood lymphocytes showing the diploid value of the DNA content.

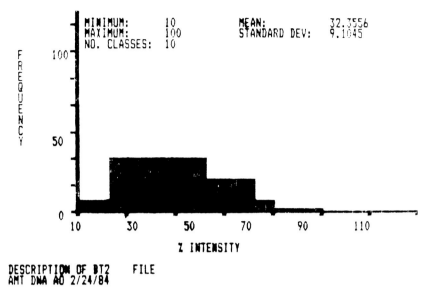

Fig. 12.7. AO-DNA histogram of breast carcinoma cells showing aneuploid DNA content (From Rosen and Mercer[40].)

archival smears which have been destained.[22,24,30,40,44] The techniques, which are well described elsewhere, are based on fluorescence measurements of nuclear DNA content on Feulgen or acridine orange-stained smears.[27,28,40]

Cytophotometric methods have the advantage of permitting the same clinical sample to be studied by quantitative cell measurements and conventional cytomorphologic criteria. Monolayers of tumor cells, as seen in imprint smears of ABC, are particularly well-suited to study by this method. The disadvantages of cytophotometry include observer bias in the subjective selection of cells to be measured, the small number of cells measured, and the relatively time-consuming and labor-intensive nature of the procedure compared to flow cytometry.[22,23] Moreover, smears with "heavy" backgrounds, as in the presence of marked tumor necrosis, inflammation, or cell products such as mucin, may be technically difficult or impossible to measure.[40]

Flow cytometry is presently more widely used than cytophotometry in the study of DNA distributions of tumors. Flow cytometry offers rapidity and the measurement of large numbers of tumor cells. This results in high resolution and the ability to assess proliferative activity by determining the percentage of cells in S phase, a measurement which appears to give important prognostic information about human tumors, including breast carcinoma.[29,32,33,36,38]

The techniques are well described elsewhere[31,37] and have been applied to a variety of clinical samples, including fresh, frozen, and paraffin-embedded tissue and NAB.[23,35,39,44] Aspirates are particularly well suited to analysis by flow cytometry, since they can be used to study small resected tissue samples without interfering with histologic interpretation and may increase the yield of nondiploid cells compared to tissue samples.[31] The disadvantage of flow cytometry is that measurements are made on cells which cannot be assessed by traditional cytomorphologic criteria.[40]

Applications

DNA ploidy levels of tumor cells reflect the nuclear DNA content. Studies of human tumors, including breast carcinoma, have shown that a correlation exists between the DNA distribution of the malignant cells and the prognosis.[21,24,34]

Investigations have suggested a relationship between DNA ploidy levels in breast carcinoma and such prognostic features as histologic grade, estrogen receptor status, and patient survival.[24,37,38] Diploid tumors tend to be associated with low histologic grade and may be associated with a more favorable disease-free survival in certain patient populations.[26,32,37,43] Some investigations have suggested a trend for DNA aneuploid tumors to be hormone receptor negative and to be associated with a less favorable disease-free period and a briefer overall patient survival time.[24,32,37,38,43]

Analysis of the DNA distribution does not appear to be useful in distinguishing benign from malignant breast tumors, since malignant tumors may show a diploid or aneuploid DNA distribution. In the literature, DNA aneuploid tumors account for 54 to 92 percent of breast carcinomas.[25,43] Reliance on the DNA distribution alone, therefore, would result in a high rate of false-negative diagnoses.[41-44] Some studies have reported rare instances of benign breast lesions showing an aneuploid DNA distribution, suggesting a small risk of false-positive diagnoses using cytometric analysis alone.[42]

The DNA distribution in breast carcinoma appears to correlate with important prognostic features. Further investigations using cytometric analysis should be pursued to establish the role of such information both in the assessment of tumor biologic aggressiveness and in the clinical management of the patient with breast cancer.

REFERENCES
High Risk Lesions

1. Azzopardi JG: *Problems in Breast Pathology.* Philadelphia, W.B. Saunders Co., 1979.

2. Broders AC: Carcinoma in situ contrasted with benign penetrating epithelium. *JAMA* 99:1670–1674, 1932.

3. Fisher ER, Sass R, Fisher B, et al: Pathologic findings from the National Surgical Adjuvant Breast Project (Protocol 6) I. Intraductal carcinoma (DCIS). *Cancer* 57:197–208, 1986.

4. Foote FW Jr, Stewart FW: Lobular carcinoma in situ: A rare form of mammary carcinoma. *Am J Pathol* 17:491–495, 1941.

5. Haagensen CD, Lane N, Lattes R, Bodian C: Lobular neoplasia (so-called lobular carcinoma in situ) of the breast. *Cancer* 42:737–769, 1978.

6. Hutter RVP: The management of patients with lobular carcinoma in situ of the breast. *Cancer* 53:798–802, 1984.

7. Kline TS: *Handbook of Fine Needle Aspiration Biopsy Cytology,* 2nd ed. New York, Churchill Livingstone, 1988.

8. Kline TS, Lundy J, Lozowski M: Monoclonal antibody B72.3: An adjunct for evaluation of "suspicious" aspiration biopsy cytology from the breast. *Cancer* (in press).

9. Lagios MD, Westdahl PR, Margolin FR, Rose MR: Duct carcinoma in situ. Relationship of extent of noninvasive disease to the frequency of occult invasion, multicentricity, lymph node metastases and short-term treatment failures. *Cancer* 50:1309–1314, 1982.

10. Lambird PA, Shelley WM: The spatial distribution of lobular in situ mammary carcinoma; implications for size and site of breast biopsy. *JAMA* 210:689–693, 1969.

11. Lattes R: Lobular neoplasia (lobular carcinoma in situ) of the breast—a histological entity of controversial clinical significance. Pathol Res Pract 166:415–429, 1980.

12. McDivitt RW, Hutter RVP, Foote FW Jr, Stewart FW: In situ lobular carcinoma. A prospective follow-up study indicating cumulative patient risks. *JAMA* 201:82–86, 1967.

13. Page DL, Anderson TJ: *Diagnostic Histopathology of the Breast.* Edinburgh, Churchill Livingstone, 1987.

14. Page DL, Dupont WD, Rogers LW, Rados MS: Atypical hyperplastic lesions of the female breast. *Cancer* 55:2698–2708, 1985.

15. Rosen PP: Lobular carcinoma in situ: Recent clinicopathologic studies at Memorial Hospital. *Pathol Res Pract* 166:430–455, 1980.

16. Rosen PP, Lieberman PH, Braun DW Jr, Kosloff C, Adair F: Lobular carcinoma in situ of the breast; detailed analysis of 99 patients with average follow-up of 24 years. *Am J Surg Pathol* 2:225–251, 1978.

17. Rosner D, Bedwani RN, Vana J, Baker HW, Murphy GP: Noninvasive breast carcinoma. Results of a national survey by the American College of Surgeons. *Ann Surg* 192:139–147, 1980.

18. Schuh ME, Nemoto T, Penetrante RB, Rosner D, Dao TL: Intraductal carcinoma; analysis of presentation, pathologic findings, and outcome of disease. *Arch Surg* 121:1303–1307, 1986.

19. Silverstein MJ, Rossner RJ, Gierson ED, et al: Axillary lymph node dissection for intraductal breast carcinoma—is it indicated? *Cancer* 59:1819–1824, 1987.

20. Wellings SR, Jensen HM, Marcum RG: An atlas of subgross pathology of the human breast with special reference to possible precancerous lesions. *J Natl Cancer Inst* 55:231–271, 1975.

DNA Distribution In Breast Carcinoma

21. Atkin B, Mattison G, Baker MC: Comparison of the DNA content and chromosome number of fifty human tumors. *Br J Cancer* 20:87–101, 1966.

22. Auer G, Tribukait B: Comparative single cell and flow DNA analysis in aspiration biopsies from breast carcinomas. *Acta Pathol Microbiol Scand (A)* 88:355–358, 1980.

23. Auer GU, Askensten U, Erharot K, Fallenius A, Zetterberg A: Comparison between slide and flow cytophotometric DNA measurements in breast tumors. *Anal Quant Cytol Histol* 9:138–146, 1987.

24. Auer GU, Caspersson TO, Wallgren AS: DNA content and survival in mammary carcinoma. *Anal Quant Cytol* 2:161–165, 1980.

25. Bedrossian CWM, Raber M, Barlogie B: Flow cytometry and cytomorphology in primary resectable breast cancer. *Anal Quant Cytol* 3:112–116, 1981.

26. Berryman IL, Harvey JM, Sterrett GF, Papadimitriou JM: The nuclear DNA content of human breast carcinoma. Associations with clinical stage, axillary lymph node status, estrogen receptor status and outcome. *Anal Quant Cytol Histol* 9:429–434, 1987.

27. Boquoi E, Krebs S, Kreuzer G: Feulgen-DNA-cytophotometry on mammary tumor cells from aspiration biopsy smears. *Acta Cytol* 19:326–329, 1975.

28. Cornelisse CJ, Tanke HJ, de Koning H, de la Riviere GB: DNA ploidy analysis and cytologic examination of sorted cell populations from human breast tumors. *Anal Quant Cytol* 5:173–183, 1983.

29. Dressler LG, Seamer LC, Owens MA, Clark GM, Mcguire WL: DNA flow cytometry and prognostic factors in 1331 frozen breast cancer specimens. *Cancer* 61:420–427, 1988.

30. Fossa SD, Marton PF, Knudsen OS, et al: Nuclear Feulgen DNA content and nuclear size in human breast carcinoma. *Hum Pathol* 13:626–630, 1982.

31. Greenebaum E, Koss LG, Sherman AB, Elequin F: Comparison of needle aspiration and solid biopsy technics in the flow cytometric study of DNA distributions of surgically resected tumors. *Am J Clin Pathol* 82:559–564, 1984.

32. Hedley DW, Rugg CA, Ng ABP, Taylor IW: Influence of cellular DNA content on disease-free survival of stage II breast cancer patients. *Cancer Res* 44:5395–5398, 1984.

33. Hedley DW, Rugg CA, Gelber RD: Association of DNA index and S-phase fraction with prognosis of nodes positive early breast cancer. *Cancer Res* 47:4729–4735, 1987.

34. Hemstreet GP, West SS, Weems WL, et al: Quantitative fluorescence measurements of AO-stained normal and malignant bladder cells. *Int J Cancer* 31:577–585, 1983.

35. Levack PA, Mullen P, Anderson TJ, Miller WR, Forrest APM: DNA analysis of breast tumor fine needle aspirates using flow cytometry. *Br J Cancer* 56:643–646, 1987.

36. McDivitt RW, Stone KR, Craig RB, et al: A proposed classification of breast cancer based on kinetic information. Derived from a comparison of risk factors in 168 primary operable breast cancers. *Cancer* 57:269–276, 1986.

37. Olszewski W, Darzykiewicz Z, Rosen PP, Schwartz MK, Melamed MR: Flow cytometry of breast carcinoma: I. Relation of DNA ploidy level to histology and estrogen receptor status. *Cancer* 48:980–984, 1981.

38. Olszewski W, Darzykiewicz Z, Rosen PP, Schwartz MK, Melamed MR: Flow cytometry of breast carcinoma: II. Relation of tumor cell cycle distribution to histology and estrogen receptor. *Cancer* 48:985–988, 1981.

39. Remvikos Y, Magoelenat H, Zajdela A: DNA flow cytometry applied to fine needle sampling of human breast cancer. *Cancer* 61:1629–1634, 1988.

40. Rosen S, Mercer WE: Cytophotometry of breast carcinoma: Acridine-orange DNA microfluorimetry with Giemsa counterstain. *Anal Quant Cytol Histol* 7:159–162, 1985.

41. Sprenger E, Ulrich H, Schöndorf H: The diagnostic value of cell-nuclear DNA determination in aspiration cytology of benign and malignant lesions of the breast. *Anal Quant Cytol* 1:29–36, 1979.

42. Spyratos F, Briffod M, Gentile A, et al: Flow cytometric study of DNA distribution in cytopunctures of benign and malignant breast lesions. *Anal Quant Cytol Histol* 9:485–494, 1987.

43. Thorud E, Fossa SD, Vaage S, et al: Primary breast cancer. Flow cytometric DNA pattern in relation to clinical and histopathologic characteristics. *Cancer* 57:808–811, 1986.

44. Zajicek J, Caspersson T, Jackobsson P, et al: Cytologic diagnosis of mammary tumors from aspiration biopsy smears. Comparison of cytologic and histologic findings in 2,111 lesions and diagnostic use of cytophotometry. *Acta Cytol* 14:370–376, 1970.

Index

Page numbers in italics refer to illustrations